FITTING IN

THE MASK OF HEALTH

FITTING IN

THE MASK OF HEALTH

ALEXANDRE CARNEIRO

Certified Health and Training
Specialist - Nutritionist

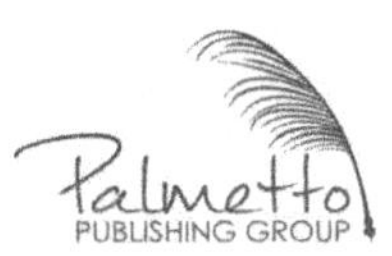

Palmetto Publishing Group
Charleston, SC

For information regarding special discounts for bulk purchases, please contact
Palmetto Publishing Group at Info@PalmettoPublishingGroup.com.

ISBN-13: 978-1-64111-030-3
ISBN-10: 1-64111-030-9

TABLE OF CONTENTS

PREFACE

Everyone has a story. This is mine. I don't know if it was all the Jean Claude Van Damme movies or Japanese cartoons I watched growing up, but something about being bigger and more muscular was appealing to me. By the age of eighteen, I had arrived in the United States ready to pursue my degree in kinesiology. I knew that I had to take advantage of the time I was given in the land of opportunities to build myself a name and legacy. Isn't that what every foreigner wants? An opportunity to achieve their own American Dream? My vision was to become someone others would recognize, respect, and seek if they wanted to learn about building a strong and bigger physique. With years of discipline, I transformed from the skinny foreigner teen I was in college to the first Latin American to achieve pro status with the International Fitness and Bodybuilding Organization (IFBB) in the physique division; to multiple international magazine covers, ads, sponsorships, television spots, a top ten contender in the world-renowned Mr. Olympia competition, and so much more. I had achieved my dreams and more. The world felt like mine to take, but as the saying goes, be careful what you wish for. I had everything I had ever wished for, but felt empty inside.

The transformation that took me years to build only focused on the external; it created a shell that I used to protect myself from life itself. While others admired my looks, I started to despise myself for not creating a healthy, balanced human. As years went by I started to notice a trend that was becoming more and more common in society, one where people only focused on taking care of the outside. The media places more of an emphasis on how people should look in order to have a happier life than how they should *feel*. Makes sense; we are judged daily on our exteriors, and we then wear a mask to showcase an illusion of health. In addition to the mask we wear outside for others to see, we wear one for ourselves to hide from who we truly are. We spend so much time on social media looking at what others are doing and how they look like, that we don't realize when we've lost sense of our surrounding circles and who we are influenced by. Those accounts we closely follow influence us more than ever. We start to create a reality in our minds of what our lives should be, based on looks and materialism, and we stop appreciating the current things we've already achieved—and those we love. We absorb the energy of those little screens, and surround ourselves only with unreality.

I was part of this epidemic problem as I promoted this image of health, when in reality, what I was projecting was far from the truth. We live now in a society where millions will do what it takes to fit into a culture of projected perfection. Teens watching hours of their favorite social media star who looks like young Hercules start thinking that it's the way they should look in order to be happy and successful in life. Sadly, many will do whatever it takes to obtain those physical attributes, and risk their health the same way I did for a vain purpose. I want to explore with you the concept that true health is slowly disappearing, and vain ideals are taking its place. False realities, Photoshop, and self-doubts from the models themselves are posted on a daily basis trying to influence you into believing what they want you to believe and feel.

I want you to understand that your power to become who you want to be has nothing to do with how low your body fat is, or whether you have the perfect body. Finally, I also want to share with you my journey that started this entire book. I want you to know the truth of what it took to be one of the best in an industry that consumed my life and distorted my vision of reality. Most importantly, I want to give you the resources and share the steps to gaining control of your motivation for you to apply in your life and health. For years I wore the mask of health on my face pretending to live a healthy lifestyle, but mentally, spiritually, and physically it was all a façade. Let me share with you the best tactics to feel motivated, to find your fitness, and start the journey for you to be in the best shape both inside and outside.

INTRODUCTION

Those who think they have no time for healthy eating . . .
will sooner or later have to find time for illness.

—Edward Stanley

Our lives are shaped by our experiences. They create our character, personalities, ethics, and everything we are today. Without experiences, we wouldn't really live. My life is a series of experiences that primarily surround one subject: fitness. For what to so many is simply a hobby—or just a tedious activity—to me, it has been my life. Because of it, I can share with you my thoughts and views, and I can explain the direction the wellness world has been shaping itself to be.

I'm going to start by asking you one question out of what I feel are the most important questions I'll be asking throughout the book. When you think about health, wellness, and fitness, what comes to mind? What images and thoughts pop into your brain? Green smoothies and detox teas? Images of strong muscles and tight midsections? Bright, neon-colored clothes? A bright white room with a young woman in perfect balance, practicing yoga? The media bombards us with what they want to sell, and what their idea of wellness should be for you. But does that truly improve your habits and motivate you to go on a journey of fitness? Or is it just an illusion they're selling?

Fitness comes in several forms and shapes, yet it still feels like you have to look a certain way in order to fit those parameters. Why do even the soda commercials and fast-food chains still use the average weight, standard-sized models for their ads, promoting this image of happy people eating and drinking their products, when in reality we know it's their products that are causing the spike in obesity and diabetes in children and adults today? How can you feel like you fit within the parameters of what you should look like in order to be happy when what you are currently doesn't match those standards? This constantly makes you seek something you don't yet have in life: the perfect body. The media is telling you to be happy—drink this, eat that, or be part of this specific activity to fit in. But the people who eat, drink, or are part of those activities don't look anything like the people routinely displayed in most ads.

From the world-renowned Muscle Beach in Venice California to the lyrics—and the unforgettable scene—of James Brown's "Living in America" from Rocky IV, the US has always been the center of the world when it comes to sports and fitness. Students around the entire globe dream from an early age to be able to be given the chance to study and earn a degree here. Why do you think an eighteen-year-old Brazilian teenager with a dream of becoming the next fitness phenomenon came to live here? Because this truly is the land of opportunity for those who work and seek success. Throughout my eleven years living in the US, I've had phenomenal opportunities, some given to me, and several I created myself. I have had opportunities I know I would never get anywhere else in the world. Such was the reason I kept pushing myself further and further with my body to be the best I could be.

Throughout my selfish journey of wanting to be "perfect," and wanting to create my own American Dream, I realized how far from health and wellness I got. But it was only through that realization that my mind opened in terms of what I was doing, and what that same marketing was telling others to do as well. The more I worried about my next competition, photoshoot, or appearance, the more I forgot about the true meaning of being internally and physically healthy. Looking good was all that mattered, but I was not aware of the side effects I was generating for myself. On top of that, I portrayed to others a perfect life; one on social media that would attract thousands and thousands of fans who wanted to be me, live like me, and act like me. It was only years later that I realized it, and asked myself, "What am I doing? In what world is anything that I am doing contributing to better health for me and those who follow me? Am I only concerned about how many likes, shares, and comments a picture gets? What about the message I'm sending?

Life is balance: true and false, good and evil, healthy and the illusion of healthy. Everything I was doing was an illusion; an illusion of health, an illusion of happiness, and an illusion of life. Was I the only one living this sort of life? Had we in the fitness industry pretty much become mannequins, displaying a life of health to others but in reality feeling like an empty shell of a person? Had we forgotten the roles as health ambassadors to pass on purposeful messages that would actually improve other's lives through exercise? Or were we just all robots trying to sell something via our bodies and pictures? Was I, along with thousands of others, sending the message that health and happiness came only from the external, physical body?

I will teach you how to regain the power you need to reach your own happiness, your own fitness goals, and truly obtain the body and health you've been seeking in balance. I want you to understand how your brain works and why you have created these barriers you, yourself, don't understand—or potentially even know about—and why they are there in first place. Allow me and my book to give you the power and knowledge to understand why it is that some have it easy when it comes to creating healthy habits, and why, for some, it's like trying to figure out a calculus equation. The principles you will learn here can be applied to any aspect of your life so that you may truly find your happiness. Read, think, write down, process, and apply.

CHAPTER 1

COMING TO THE UNITED STATES

As you know, I'm an immigrant. I came over here as an immigrant, and what gave me the opportunities, what made me to be here today, is the open arms of Americans. I have been received. I have been adopted by America.
—Arnold Schwarzenegger

What is your dream? What's the one thing you want most of all? Money? Fame? Both? We seem to always want the one thing that we currently don't have in our lives, and when we get it we still want more. It's human nature. We sadly also forget the experiences and hardships it took to get those initial things. I've had the chance to work with CEOs, celebrities, and many others who have had it all and yet still weren't happy. You name it: beautiful significant others, a lot of money, international real estate, and power. That eternal quest for the thing that's missing never ends, because we focus so much on what we can or should get that we never appreciate what we already have.

So many incredible clients have crossed my path, and they all knew that they couldn't buy a healthier lifestyle. They'd have to sweat and grind weekly if they wanted to see any internal changes to their lives. They would have to apply effort and have to put the down the drinks in order to change the one thing money couldn't buy. Surgery can only modify the external, but actual health can't be bought that way overnight. Sure, having money means one can afford better treatments, drugs, and healthcare, but what if you could just avoid that altogether by investing in your health daily to avoid all those hassles? Would you do it? Avoiding pills and feeling naturally energized, you could be ready to take on anything life throws at you. With over a decade spent working as a trainer, you'd be surprised how few times someone came up and said to me, "I want to be healthier" or "I want to live longer." Isn't that what we should all be desiring for ourselves? Is the new American Dream no longer *actual* success, but just the image of it? Do we all just want to fit within the parameters of what marketing makes us feel we should be?

• • •

It was 2006 when I landed in the United States. Colorado was the state in which I was going to spend the next few years of my life. I was thrilled to leave and start a new chapter in my life. I can't really describe how I felt; I only remember feeling anxious. Believe it or not, I actually wanted classes to start. I wanted to experience this whole new freedom I would get that would allow me to create my future. You'd think after seeing my dorm and meeting my new roommates that I would want to meet local girls and see the town, but my first question to my roommates was, "Have you guys checked out the rec center here yet?" I was excited to see where I would be training for the next few years.

I already had a vision created in my mind as to how I would spend my time and how I wanted my body to look like. Of course, like any person, my expectations were way unrealistic: big pecs, tight abs, and big arms, etc. That would impress the girls and get me closer to landing a cover, I would think to myself. I would go to my classes during the day, train hard in the evening, and study at night. That was the ideal life for me. At that time I didn't know much about nutrition. I only knew the basics, but it was enough to motivate me into learning more. Working out was easy; just lift heavy things up, and then put them down.

Throughout my years in college, all of my friendships were made inside the rec center. People I recognized on campus were individuals I'd met at the rec center; not people I'd met because of late-night parties, or even people in my classes. In fact, I didn't go out much to parties. People would also recognize me and say, "I see you at the rec center a lot. What's your name?" I guess you could call me a little bit of an outcast. Getting drunk and feeling hangovers were not on my list of priorities. Skip forward almost eleven years later, and they still aren't. If I couldn't work out, then it wasn't a successful day, so why compromise that with alcohol the night before? Years later, however, this mindset developed into an unbalanced, obsessive life, a life I didn't expect to be so out of sync with the real world.

At that time, though, I felt it was the right thing to do in order to be successful. I associated parties with alcohol and dumb college kids pressuring me to drink. Instead, I should have seen the socializing aspect to it. Today I regret not having a bit more fun in college, or enjoying the college experience more. Every decision I made then, however, led me to write this book, so never regret what you didn't do in your past—only regret the things you don't do in your future.

At the age of twenty, I met my ex-wife. For the next two years as I was finishing school, she and I would spent as much time as possible together on the weekends. She lived about an hour away from me, but we made it work, and of course we would work out together on the weekends. I learned to enjoy having another person in my life, as I'd always been on my own since I arrived in the U.S, and I hadn't ever bonded with anyone else. Dating was also not on my list of things to do, so when I met her and our lives started growing together, that was a new experience I was learning to enjoy. I liked that she would switch a few things around during her day so she could fit in a good workout with me. It made me feel like she cared about it, too.

Over time, I understood that one should never impose their own lifestyle and habits onto another person. It will make them resent you and dislike you as an individual. In several relationships after my divorce, I was told I was controlling, and I realized that tendency came from my years of being lonely before my marriage. I wanted others to live by my rules and habits. There was no other way to do things but my own. I did that with my ex-wife a lot, and over time she slowly started to resent me for it. She was a good woman, and to please me she would do things my way—but one day, enough was enough.

Eventually this lifestyle created a lot of problems in our relationship, and it ended up being a large reason for our divorce. To be honest, I was not the best husband. I spent the majority of the time thinking about myself, my goals, and my body. I didn't listen to anyone else but myself. At that age and in that phase of my life, I had already become too self-centered, and anyone who tried to get me to see a different viewpoint of what fitness, health, and life itself was about, was wrong. My own parents, who always wanted what was best for me, tried giving me advice about marriage and I never took it. I don't regret having that mindset back in the day, as it established a foundation for success in the industry I was involved in. I had a goal and a vision and no one would take that away from me.

As I look back, I know what my mistakes were. Failing is just learning from your experiences so that in the future you fail in different ways until you get it right, and eventually learn from the past. Hopefully we all make the mistakes we have to make in order to learn and grow from them. In a way, I'm happy these things all happened at an earlier age so that today I can just look back and be thankful they didn't happen later in life. Thinking back and wishing we could have done things differently only eats us alive, yet learning from them and avoiding them in the future means true growth.

The land of opportunity truly was everything I had wished for: well-equipped gyms, updated literature to learn from, supplement stores, twenty-four-hour fitness facilities . . . it was all there. I remember years later reading Arnold Schwarzenegger's autobiography, and his explanation of what his first encounters and adventures here in the US were like. His words made me feel like I knew exactly what he had gone through, as I, too, was amazed at all the incredible facilities and things people had access to here. Back in the day there wasn't much need for Wi-Fi, since most phones didn't use data to play music or watch videos, yet in 2006 my rec center already had these incredible resources for students to use.

Things so small seemed so incredible. The tools were laid out, and I couldn't' believe how happy and blessed I was to be given the chance to be in this country. Interestingly, something I've observed over the course of my many years living here is that many Americans don't value the small things they have daily; they take them for granted. Just to give you an idea: a five-pound tub of protein powder in the US currently averages anywhere between forty-five and sixty dollars depending on the brand, the location where it's being sold, etc. Outside of the US, that same product would most likely be a hundred dollars or more. The small things I myself took for granted after living here for so long are the things I'm reminded to appreciate every time I leave the country for work, and I remember how lucky I am to live here.

Hard labor is considered tremendously more valuable here than anywhere outside of this country. A personal trainer in Brazil on average makes anywhere between six and nine dollars an hour, a rate which in many states is lower than minimum wage. There isn't much opportunity after that. Here, a personal trainer has the chance to easily make triple that amount—or more. So you see, for many foreigners living in the US, living conditions are better in all possible aspects than they would be living back home. Wanting to fit in in American culture is just a long-lost dream for so many outside of this country.

Becoming a citizen was a no-brainer for me. I knew after just a few months of living here that this is where I wanted to stay, and that I would work hard to build a name for myself and build something for which I would be remembered. Even though I did come from a great family who provided me with everything, I had to work countless hours on my programs, my websites, and other tools I used to grow my business. These things were not handed to me. Nothing was done overnight, or quickly. We currently live in a society where people want things done fast and easily; that's the norm these days. But fast and easy are words that will never be associated with anyone who's made it far in life. To ask for something to be fast and easy is to ask for something to also end fast and easy.

Fitness is a universal language, similar to math. When you go to a gym, the dumbbells are the same, the barbells are the same, and anywhere in the world you go train, two-hundred-pound squats feel amazing no matter what. For **many**, the gym is a place to socialize, a place to meditate, and somewhere to release stress. No matter the reason anyone goes, the gym is there for those seeking to improve themselves in one way or another. That's the mindset I did not have when I was in my early twenties and had just graduated from college. I believed everyone had to lift weights, and only weights. Yoga and Pilates were for hippies; cycling and any type of endurance sport were for people who couldn't put on muscle; powerlifters and strongmen were just fat individuals who were pretending to be fit; and anything related to stretching should be done elsewhere than a gym.

My mentality was extremely close-minded, and health was definitely not on my mind. Most twenty-year-old young men feel indestructible, and I was no different. My only goal was to get big—as big as possible—no matter what. I was eating anything and everything in sight, no matter if it was junk food or home-cooked food. All I cared about was watching the number on the scale go up. I believe this is where my journey that led me to a vain, empty shell of a life began—a journey I originally thought I was destined to take—but I wasn't aware of who it would turn me into, and what it would do to my health.

Think about the following things.

- What do you desire out of this life? Write down your short- and long-term goals, and place them somewhere where you will be sure to look at them daily. (I recommend on top of your alarm clock.)
- Write down three to five things you have accomplished already in your lifetime of which you are proud. Never forget that you've already come a long way in life just by living it. If you can't name three to five accomplishments, then go back to the first bullet point and add those as goals you desire to achieve.
- Do you have a vision of how you want your health and life to be? Visualizing your success and how you will get there is the first step.

- Are you open to new ideas? Remember that two plus two equals four—but so does three plus one. Be open to different ways of solving your current problems.

CHAPTER 2

FITTING IN MY OWN SKIN

In a crowded marketplace, fitting in is a failure. In a busy marketplace, not standing out is the same as being invisible.

—Seth Godin

Many have asked me why I chose to live in Colorado. A decade later I still get asked, "Isn't California, Florida—or at least New York—better for your industry?" These locations are indeed better for the fitness industry, as they have more people spending and investing money. Additionally, the chance of working with celebrities and bigger companies is more likely to happen there than anywhere else. However, I wasn't going to allow my location to define my odds of being one of the best. Not only did I land one of the giants of the supplement world as my sponsor, but because of them, I have had the chance to work with companies like 24 Hour Fitness and Amazon. So don't allow your current circumstances to be one of the reasons to push you back from attaining your ultimate goals.

In the end, Colorado gave me a phenomenal education and experience, and I wouldn't be where I am today if I had not moved here. Sometimes we wonder what life would be if we'd made different choices in the past, but I can say that living here for as long as I have isn't something I question. I used to daydream a lot back in the day, and pretend what it would be like to live in different places, imagining the people I would meet or where I'd be working. I believe doing that occasionally is fine, but spending too much time in dreamland can become a bad habit, as it can lead us to think our current situation isn't good enough. Always remember that the past is the past, and the actions you took can't be undone. Worry about the changes you can make today to affect tomorrow. That's how I want you to start thinking when it comes to your daily actions regarding your health. Don't take action tomorrow when it can be done today.

By the age of twenty-one I had already won my first state bodybuilding show. I felt like all those hard hours at the gym had paid off, which meant if I wanted to be better I had to invest even more time in myself. The pats on my back and the congratulations after it was all done were fulfilling. However, two days later it was over. The only thing left were memories. Just like a drug, I needed more. I needed more of that type of attention. Uploading pictures on social media and reading the compliments was an additional boost to my ego, but it wasn't enough. I needed and wanted more.

So it was back to the drawing board, and I repeated what I had done before: eat, sleep, train, and repeat. You might wonder where in that cycle I made time for friends, time for my wife, or time for anything else. Well, there wasn't any time for those things. I had tunnel vision, and all I saw was this vision of perfection. By the age of twenty-three I already had my first fitness magazine cover, was among the top ten in the world, had sponsors, and was one of the rising stars in the fitness industry—but I was also going through my divorce.

It didn't take too much to get sucked into my own world, a world where I would wake up every morning, weigh myself, measure out my food for the day, take my supplements, and go to the gym once or twice a day. A world that involved me and only me, and that was the issue. Going through that divorce didn't make me stronger initially. In fact, I kept using my narcissistic ways to pull myself out of it. I used the gym, once again, as my drug of choice to forget the world. Inside the gym all I got were compliments, encouraging words, and "friends" who would cheer me up. Trust me, there was nothing good about going to the gym with that mindset.

I just wanted to replace my emotions of sadness with another exercise; replace all memories of what was currently happening to me with another set of reps. Working out released a lot of endorphins that made me feel good about myself; being in the gym was probably the only place I could seek happiness, since at home I didn't have any of that. At the gym I had control, but at home I didn't. In the process of hiding my emotions I even a broke my right hand, and I only had myself to blame, as I had lost control of my emotions one day and punched through a panel of glass in the kitchen. Dumbest moment of my life, I can admit. I was so embarrassed that I had lost all control over my feelings. I had everything I had ever wanted to achieve since I'd first stepped foot off the plane that had brought me here, and yet I had lost the only family I had in this country. It was a lonely phase in my life.

While this phase continued, I kept making more and more mistakes without realizing it. It was only years later, after being in my current relationship, that I realized my image was only a mask I was wearing to impress others with my accomplishments. I don't regret working hard, but I do regret not balancing that hard work with real life. It took several years for me to realize that my vanity was masking my health, and not making me a better individual.

Hell, I wasn't making anyone better. Additionally, I also realized that if I couldn't be mentally balanced to help myself, then how would I preach the importance of that to my clients?

Fast-forward a few years later and I have sadly seen many others going that same route in life: people immersing themselves in their narcissistic ways because of some fitness competition or new job, losing track of everything around them. Some stories are worse than mine, with those individuals in their mid-forties still concerned with how the world sees and judges them. One of the worst side effects of this type of lifestyle is that all family and friends take a back seat. Health comes third, if it's considered at all.

I've witnessed so many divorces that came about as a result of an industry that prioritizes vanity over everything else. Couples I observed walking into the gym together, months later couldn't even stand each other's company. Narcissism and ego tend to do awful things. Later, I did understand why my ex-wife felt like leaving me. Sometimes we aren't supposed to understand the current events happening in our lives until moments, years, or maybe decades later. Our minds transform with time, and understanding certain events requires that transformation in order to fully grasp what occurred.

When everything and everyone reminds you of something painful, then naturally you just want to leave the current environment and start fresh, start from scratch and begin working in an entirely new industry with a new lifestyle. What would I do? Honestly I had no idea, but the competitive fitness industry left such a bad taste in my mouth that I didn't want to associate myself with anyone in it. No matter what gym I would find myself going to, there would always be someone who would recognize me and ask me when I'd be back on stage competing. I never truly grasped why others were so interested in knowing why I wouldn't step on stage again, or what actions I was going to take in the future. It made me think I was an object or source of entertainment for them.

Later I would question those who wanted to enter that world, and I would ask them why they wanted to do so. I would share a shorter version of my story so I could enlighten them what that world was all about. Nevertheless, I felt like it didn't change their minds—not even a bit. I wasn't trying to convince them to stop, but I wanted to share with them the reality of it and give them a few things to consider. But just like a younger version of myself, those people wouldn't listen to any of my advice.

I believe social media has made things worse, to some extent. A lot of the athletes who compete make their lives seem glorious—majestic, even—through their pictures and videos. What most people never realize, is that just like the bodies those athletes created to showcase, their social media, too, was a false portrayal of life—all done with the purpose of selling a fitness program in an attempt to make others think they, too, can be like that if they just buy whatever's being sold. At first I believed that giving advice to those who were entering that world would be hypocritical of me, as I had lived and competed in so many shows. Who was I to give my perspective of the industry after I had left it? Shouldn't others have to experience it, too, so they could make up their own minds?

But as time went by, I realized that my story had many duplicates. I had several competitors from all parts of the world who knew my story and contacted me; they wanted to know how to get their loved ones back, how to stabilize and balance their lives, how to simply get back to loving fitness itself. To those who wanted to train with me to get ready for a physique or bikini competition, I would even offer a different route for their fitness journey. I would lower my prices and explain that I would work with them to achieve their goals without the pressure of having to step on stage, or even having to feel the pressure of reaching a weight-loss goal by a specific date. Let me tell you this: When a date is added to the equation and you have to get into a certain shape and look a certain way by X date, pressure is added. People now will do anything to win, and the original intentions of dropping weight slowly are rushed to yet maximum point.

The comparison game starts, as well. Folks would send me pictures of other athletes on social media they followed, and ask me how they could achieve that look or get a specific body part to be a certain way. They wanted to look exactly like someone else. Unfortunately, I did not own a genetic mutation machine that would transform people's bodies into other people's bodies, so additionally, I now had to play the role of psychologist, and explain to them that we're all different, that it's okay to be yourself, and not your favorite social-media influencer. No matter how hard you work and how dedicated you are, you'll never be able to be or look like someone else. I did guarantee they could look like their own best version of themselves, though.

That wasn't acceptable for so many of them, however, and they would seek out other coaches until someone out there, in exchange for a certain amount of money, would tell them it was possible. This image of perfection was a must, and I knew exactly how they felt. That's the only way they could explain to themselves the hours spent in the gym, the money spent in preparation, and the overall time they put into it. What so many fail to realize, is that you never know what goes on behind the curtains of someone else's life. You can't guess if the person is using illegal substances to achieve that body, if they've had surgery, if the picture of them is photoshopped, or how many years they've already been training. There are too many factors that can affect a single picture.

Even some of the most gorgeous and physically active people still have enormous self-image issues, and need to touch up their pictures to feel satisfied. I would be impressed by the amount of women who could easily be on the cover of any magazine yet routinely doubted themselves, doubting how they looked and how they could be. The confidence portrayed on social media can be a complete lie. In fact, the need for likes, comments, and shares was a must for these people, just like it was for me. If a certain picture did not get enough attention, then the next picture had to have more cleavage, more skin, and more provocative gestures in order to bring more attention.

Attention is the name of the game, since, as humans, we crave it in one way or another. Unfortunately, it's now a global issue no one can escape from. It didn't matter if I lived in Colorado or Japan—I couldn't escape from feeling a certain way at that time. I realized already that starting fresh elsewhere was sometimes just a fast, quick fix. The long-lasting fix needed to come from internal changes.

Think about these things going forward:

- Stop thinking about the things you should have done, and start focusing your energy on the things you can do now for a better tomorrow.
- Your current circumstances don't define you. Your actions today towards your ultimate goals, do.
- Sometimes you aren't supposed to understand current events in your life until later. It will all click in due time.
- It's okay to be yourself. You have qualities that no one else may have. Be proud of your physical and mental distinctions, as those things make you unique. What you might see as a flaw, someone else may see as one of your strengths.
- Escaping your current problems with the illusion of a new life is tempting, but your problems will always follow you. It's best for you to face them, and grow stronger from them.

CHAPTER 3

LOSING BALANCE, LOSING REALITY

Health is a state of complete physical, mental and social
well-being and not merely the absence of disease or infirmity.
—World Health Organization

You might not know it, but the day we lose track of ourselves is the day we start a long journey of self-growth. I had not realized it, but the day I started this journey myself was the day I took what made me happy and turned that into a lifelong profession, a profession that required me to push my body to its max capacity. Competing was all about how you looked on stage, so there was no space for anything but perfection. I'm sure we've all heard that we should follow our passions and try to turn them into our jobs. What I did not know back then, was that my passion was to help others achieve their own lifestyle and wellness goals through nutrition and exercise—not by living inside a gym.

Working out was a hobby that I turned into a job, that I then depended on to live. How I looked was how I judged whether I was doing a good or bad job. I loved being in the gym, loved the feeling of waking up, getting things ready, and heading out to challenge myself physically. The thought of just going a few pounds heavier on the next squat, going faster, or simply knowing I would be sore the next few days because of that hard training excited me and made me want to be there in the gym. But over time, that feeling disappeared. Now I had to be in there, now I had to force myself to go do something I was no longer passionate about. Why? Because I had everything I wanted, but I didn't want to lose it, and in order not to lose that, I couldn't slack off. If version 1.0 of my body was good, then I needed to be version 2.0 of myself to further progress. Then, just like software, I would have to be better, with fewer flaws, because if software has flaws, then people don't want to use or enjoy it anymore.

I've realized there are two types of people: those who reach their goals and eventually plateau because they are comfortable being there, and those who reach their goals and strive for more. To be one of the best athletes in my industry—in the world—meant to constantly look the part. Compete and win. Be a walking trophy. This required constant dedication and attention to myself. I could not plateau or stop; otherwise, in the back of my mind I felt like it meant I had lost. We become sucked into our lives, our diets, and our training, and anyone who is even trying to show and give us love gets omitted. In fact, I have seen so many great souls transform into the ugliest human beings because of what the power of vanity had created.

Today I always ask people why they want to compete in a physique competition. I always want to know the *why* behind their goal. I want to know the reason why they need to spend hours in the gym, diet, and do illegal substances in order to look a certain way for only a few hours, to be subjected to a panel of random judges who sometimes have never exercised themselves. Most of the answers I get are lies. Even the answers these people give have a masked quality to them. It's not my purpose to ask people why they do what they do, but I do remind them that the intentions have to be so strong, that they won't give up no matter what. The feeling of being hungry all day and how it affects your every decision isn't something many think about when they imagine a perfectly sculpted six-pack. They only think of how it will feel like to take that selfie in front of the gym mirrors and share it for everyone to see. No one thinks about how hard it is to get there.

It's through that process, though, that we get lost in ourselves, that we become so self-absorbed that vanity is more important than any other aspect of our lives. The funny thing about vanity is that it only lasts for a while, and during that time when it seems like it's going to last, we fall in love with ourselves, our selfies, and what others have to say about us. We become modern versions of Narcissus, the god in Greek mythology who fell in love with his own reflection.

Have you ever thought about why the bad guys in movies become bad? Why they're the villains as opposed to the heroes? Most times it's because they had a childhood experience that affected them so deeply and strongly that they were forced to see the world differently in order to cope with whatever happened to them. But heroes, too, can have these backgrounds, and yet somehow they turn out to be good guys instead of villains. So what's the difference? What creates a villain and what creates a hero? I've always thought that villains start seeing the world differently because they want to create a reality that requires others to see the world the way they do, to sometimes feel and experience what they have. The good guys stay within society's boundaries, and as much as they wish they could change things, they don't, because they know deep down that's not the right thing.

What's this all have to do with losing balance and a sense of reality in my life? Perception. Perception is everything in life. How we perceive things around us and about ourselves is truly what defines us as beings. How we perceive any event, including tragedies, truly comes down to us. If we decide to use a tragedy to propel us to be better, then there's a lesson learned there. More importantly, how we act upon those events will further dramatically change us. The way you see the world around yourself is the way you will start molding who you are, both with yourself and others. When it comes to your health, you should start to perceive it as an attribute in your life that could bring you extreme joy or extreme pain.

You don't need great talent to start, but you do need to start somewhere. Don't wait for your health to deteriorate or cause you physical and emotional pain to begin your journey. Begin now, at this instant, and start taking care of yourself. Too many wait for their own bodies to have to tell them via pain before they start taking care of themselves; others need a wakeup call in order to start. Prevent all of that by simply taking care of yourself today. Your reality is dramatically altered by your perception of everything around you. In my case, my reality was distorted by bodies and vanity. But aren't more people today being shown a reality of physical distortion? A reality of happiness based on looks? Losing balance is easier than ever when you are shown daily on social media how you should look in order to tell you how you should feel. Who are you going to be? The hero or villain? After all, they are one in the same, and the only difference between the two is the individual's perception of reality.

In years of competing and being involved in the fitness community, my perception of people had changed, and trust me, in no way good. I felt everyone was a weakling, that anyone who didn't have discipline in their lives was simply a weak-minded individual. In my mind, if someone wanted to lose five pounds, then it was simple: Stop eating as much. Exercise. Boom! So easy! But no, people would find more excuses than solutions for themselves. They wanted to take magic pills, or try everything other than working hard. So why couldn't Jane or Joe lose five pounds? Because they were weak. They couldn't control their emotions and they had weak mindsets, which leads to weak decision-making and poor habits. That's how I used to think about others.

It's hard to share that fact with you, but that's how I viewed people in general. I had no empathy for anyone who crossed my path who said things like, "It's hard," "I'm trying," or "I wish it was easier." I'd had to walk on glass to get what I wanted, while others wanted to walk along the beach on pristine, white sand. The way I started to look at society was the same way any movie villain did. I sacrificed so much that I felt others, too, had to sacrifice the same—or more—if they wanted to achieve their physique goals or if they wanted to get anything out of life in general. I wanted others to see the world through my perspective and realize what a bunch of weaklings they were.

It was like I was a judge in one of the competitions I'd competed in. I would not only judge people on their actions, but on their physical attributes. "Good glutes, but could use more hamstring"; "Nice shoulders, but she needs more triceps to go along with that." Who was I to be judging anyone like that? If they were not in shape that meant they had no self-discipline, and were not worthy. Was this all a byproduct of being surrounded by people like myself for many years? Finally, I also didn't want to have "normal-looking" friends. I wanted to be surrounded by guys who also spent time in the gym and looked the part. I wanted to fit in with the big guys. Coolness by association, I guess.

As I analyze later why my mindset created this distortion, I sometimes think about the cartoons and movies I grew up with. After all, I learned the majority of my English by watching Saturday morning American cartoons like "Extreme Sharks," Power Rangers, and so many other action-themed shows. In movies, big guys would always surround Arnold Schwarzenegger. Watch *Predator*;

you won't see a single normal-looking guy. If you do see one, they probably died within the first hour of the movie. They were all jacked military men. I thought that fitting in with a group of buff guys was essential if I wanted to be an alpha male in our society.

I know this all sounds crazy, but it was my reality at that time, and my perspective of losing my balance. Funny enough, the guys who I'd thought at first glance were "cool"—because they had great-looking physiques—were in fact the ones who'd experienced the greatest amount of problems in their lives. Most of them couldn't pay their next month's rent, keep relationships, or function the way people do in normal living situations. I felt like it was the complete opposite of what I'd grown up watching on television and the big screen. Now when I think about it I laugh, but back in the day when we would go out I'd think to myself, "I made it. I'm one of them." They say some people are meant to enter your life at specific moments. I'm just glad they did not stick around longer than they had to.

Losing balance and your perception of reality is easy, especially in our current times. The reality today involves small screens we carry with us at all times; devices we look at more than the people who physically surround us. Next time you go to a public place or are sitting in a waiting room, count how many times people look at their phones. Or how about when people are having dinner with one another; see how many times the majority of those people are on their phones. I'm guilty of doing this on so many occasions. The events on the small screen are more rewarding than the events happening in real life. A "like" in the virtual world is more appreciated than a "like" from a loved one. Even in most gyms these days you will see a large percentage of people looking down at their phones—sadly, sometimes, for longer than the actual workout they came there to do.

We interact so much with others online that we don't interact with the people around us anymore. During my college years, social media was still growing. I want to say MySpace was the most popular platform at the time. Instagram hadn't been invented yet. I remember spending hours on the computer trying to build my fan page on Facebook. Today I use that same fan page to give out free advice and to post a lot of free clips in order to help others. If one person learns something new on a daily basis, I'm happy and I did my job—but it did not start that way.

As I logged online and began to delete old content on that page, I realized that for years all my page truly was, in fact, was an album of selfies of me at the gym or at home. Back to back, it was all pictures of me—shirtless. I laugh at myself now, as there was no purpose to any of those pictures other than to satisfy my need for attention and reassurance. Since I wasn't getting that from my wife, I needed to feel like I was still "someone." I never in my entire life replied to any of the women who wrote to me on social media, but I definitely liked the attention I got from them. Why shouldn't I, after all?

My ex-wife was a very beautiful woman, but online I had hundreds of women who wanted to talk to me. That attention gave me reassurance; I was looking to others for emotional support, and it made me slowly forget my relationship with my wife in real life. I would easily spend five or six hours on the computer making sure my Facebook was updated, blogs were written, and that I'd created the latest content on my membership website at the time. Most nights, my ex-wife would come back home to find me still on the computer. I would not give her any love or attention. I see years later what my mistakes were, but at the time I was consumed with my social media and with competing. My reality was twisted, and my morals were not in place.

When I try to remember why I did everything I did, I always come back to one thought: When I began all of this, I knew I needed a coach for myself, someone to look at me, give me advice on my nutrition and training—basically someone to babysit me. I remember he once asked me while we were sitting in the middle of his driveway one night, "Alex, would you rather be famous or would you rather make money?" My answer at the time was, "I want to be famous, because I can turn that into money." He just smirked at me, nodded his head, and said okay. Only time can teach a person whether they're right or wrong, and in my case I was wrong. Fame did not do anything for me. If anything, it made my life complicated and annoying, as I had to deal with all the fake friends who continually hovered around me.

What I thought was important, and would bring me happiness, only brought me sadness, depression, and darkness. In a way I'm glad I lost my sense of reality at that young of an age. It's an empty life filled with illusions. No matter how old one is, the potential to create the illusion of a better life based on the imagery in other people's social media can occur if it's allowed. The problem with me was that I was unhappy with my life, although I did not know I was. If you are somewhat unhappy in your own life, in your own skin, and in your own mind, then I hope my story will help you understand that only you have the power to make the choices needed for your life to change. Living the illusion that you are happy will only create a dark sinkhole, one into which you will fall deeper and deeper, by the way.

I will share something with you that hopefully cheers you up. If you *do* fall down that sinkhole, there's always a rope that will pull you up. That rope will come in the shape of different events, friends, loved ones, and most importantly, your ways of thinking. On any given occasion, you will always have the internal power to drive yourself to the gym, to eat better, and to create the habits you need maintain that will satisfy your definition of happiness and wellness.

- Being a better version of yourself requires that you also learn how to balance all-important attributes of your life. Don't improve things in one area and neglect another. Doing so could affect your loved ones—or you—and it could later become a bigger problem than the one you had originally.

- Be the hero in your life, and perceive health as a good deed that you are doing for yourself. There's no true reason you can't control the outcome of all your actions that affect your wellbeing today.

- Life is too short to give a small screen more attention than those people around you. Don't create a reality where your phone is what you prioritize over your time spent with others.

- You are a living person with the capacity to chance any circumstances in your life. When you are sad, angry, anxious, etc., remember that there's always a rope to pull you out of that sinkhole. Sometimes you might not know what that rope actually is, but it will reveal itself when it's the right time.

CHAPTER 4

THE ADDICTION I CREATED

"We are addicted to our thoughts. We cannot change anything if we cannot change our thinking."
—Santosh Kalwar

Did you know that the word "health" means "wholeness"? With that said, to be complete—to feel whole—would mean that you are balanced in both mind and body. Would you then consider yourself healthy if either one of those isn't balanced? Can you have a healthy mind but an unhealthy body? Or have a healthy body and an unhealthy mind? Think about that, as one affects the other in multiple ways. My unbalance began with an unhealthy mindset, which led to an unhealthy body. It was a symbiotic relationship where I constantly fed polluted thoughts to my mind.

Whenever you think of an addiction, you probably don't tend to think of anything positive. It's one of those words that, for decades, has always had negative connotations and is associated with things like drugs, alcohol, and smoking. Have you ever heard anyone say, "Yeah, he's addicted to happiness!"? Me neither! That *can* happen, but you're unlikely to hear of it. Even if someone said, "He's addicted to fitness"—that doesn't seem too positive of a statement. Any addiction simply means there is a lack of true balance in life. It's different when someone actually enjoys doing something and spends time being involved in it than it is when someone spends the entire day thinking about it, and all their other actions are affected by it.

It's rare to find an addiction that doesn't impact those around the individual who has the problem. The energy feels sucked out of things. However, in the fitness community most would say that's normal; that's the way it must be done in order to truly succeed; that you must be truly obsessed with that lifestyle in order to be the best. That's what I started believing from day one. With most addictions, the individual will most likely not admit to having one, and they won't be happy if you call them out on it. It's also common for individuals to not even know they have an addiction; I surely didn't think I had one. The common thought process is that if it's not affecting others, then it must not be bad. I didn't even know I had an addiction until after years of being into it.

My divorce was just a small wakeup call, but my body giving up on me was also not enough. It was only when I realized that my mindset wasn't working to my benefit and making me a better human that I started thinking I was not okay. My next few relationships did not end well either, and I started to see a pattern: It was me. That didn't slow me down, though; even being aware of my addiction wasn't enough for me to tell myself that I needed to re-evaluate my life. For over five years, no one ever told me I had a problem; no one ever sat me down and had a serious conversation with me about what I was doing to myself. The mask I was wearing was so well placed on my face that no one could tell. Only one person would open my third eye and make me see a lot of the things that I couldn't. She put my life into perspective. Without her

I probably would still be on the same destructive path.

I've never gambled with money, but I definitely gambled with my health and my everyday mental state. Every time I would do well at a competition I would tell myself, "Maybe if I diet a bit more, change my posing, push myself more at the gym—then I'll have a better chance of winning next time." Constantly placing second or third made it easier to have this mentality, because I was always *almost* there. So I would go back to the gym, dehydrated, malnourished, and tired beyond the normal limits in order to push myself, and I was proud of it—proud that I could push beyond what normal people would think was insanity. My body would give me signs; I was constantly sick, my joints and muscles always ached, and I had a hard time sleeping.

One time, I clearly remember fainting on the treadmill because my blood glucose level was too low and I had been training for about three hours straight. But hey! I looked awesome: striations all over my body, a "perfect" six-pack, and phenomenal symmetry. I felt like I had the body of a god with the mental capacity of a goldfish. This state of pushing myself until I was miserable kept going on for five or six years straight. For any normal person this sounds idiotic. It was! I was competing to win a fifteen dollar plastic trophy and to potentially get some recognition, but that was what everyone in the industry was doing—and still does!

So inside my head, that was the standard. If I wanted to fit in and be the best at what I did, then my body would have to simply get stronger, and not bother me with signs of overtraining. That was the norm for all of us, and let me share with you what traditionally happens backstage at physique shows. All the competitors would meet up backstage and discuss what their diets had been like leading up to that point. I clearly remember two things: either the competitors would lie and tell each other dieting was a breeze, or it was all about how brutal and extreme their diets were. I remember feeling upset at those who had shared their stories who claimed how easy it had been to achieve a body-fat percentage in the single digits. I knew those were lies, and that they were just trying to play it cool.

If anything, I would rather hear the struggles it took them to get where they were; that would be more human. Might I also remind you that most of these guys would be the ones you would also see later on the cover of magazines promoting how to eat and train to get in shape for the summer—when they were basically starving their bodies to get to that point. But to be human was the least of what we wanted. We wanted to stand out, and if anything else, be like super-humans. The time backstage was to scare and intimidate the fellow competitors who were going to be onstage with you. The whole point would be to make one of the guys look superior so in the last few minutes before stepping onstage, the others would start questioning themselves. I knew half of them were lying because their girlfriends would come up to me at the venues later and ask me how I did it—how was I able to stay in a normal relationship. They would say they were going borderline crazy with their boy-friends, and their crazy, competitive lifestyles.

I would tell them I'd already been through some bad times, but that communication was the key. Usually I would sit in a corner and listen to some music, and try to keep my nerves down. At that point I had done everything I could do, and it was just the time to showcase all the hard work I'd done for months to prepare for the competition. I would always think about all the sacrifices, the hours of hard work, and everything else I did to get on that stage. Often tears would come to my eyes, as I knew how much I had invested in that one moment to come. But the addiction—and its conse-quences—weren't over.

When you are done—when you've earned your trophies (if you placed) and you're headed back home—your body is still in a state of survival. The dehydration process athletes go through can truly cause problems. In fact, some athletes have passed away from the cumulative effects of having taken strong pharmaceutical diuretics for decades. From edemas to having to go to the hospital and getting an IV, if the athletes didn't know what they were doing, then it could cause serious issues.

That's not even the end of it, either. Here's some extra fun that comes with having that starving, dehydrated body: What do you think most competitors do in the days following a competition? They binge eat until they can't even move! Before that happens, though, most of the photo shoots will have been completed, most of the selfies shared throughout the year will have been saved, and most of the ads promoting any type of healthy lifestyle will have concluded. I've heard stories from competitors who tell me they easily gained back thirty pounds or more in just a few weeks. For months we would starve our bodies, and pretty much only feed it certain foods.

When you take away all the junk food and all the sweets, those things are all you crave. It's this typical situation: If I ask you not to think of the color red, what would you do? Most people immediately do just that. Let's take that example and apply it to food. For the next three or four months, we would be banned from eating certain foods. What do you think happens after you're done? Trust me, you're not going to go eat a cucumber and lettuce salad. I've done this myself several times. I remember after one of my shows in Vegas that I didn't even bother slowly rehydrating. I went straight to one of those mall vendors and got me a vodka, a Slurpee with four shots.

After reading that, I'm sure you think I'm an idiot. I agree with you there. The sugar and alcohol combined got me drunk and nauseated for almost two days because I didn't rehydrate my body when it needed it the most. On top of that, I remember going on a sugar frenzy and eating twenty Pop-Tarts. You might think I'm exaggerating, but I'm not. I had twenty Pop-Tarts and a few Snickers bars. I learned my lesson—trust me. As you are reading this, you might also think I was an oddity, one of just a few competitors who did this. Oh, no! I've heard stories that are identical to mine, but worse.

The irony of spending months to lose weight at all costs only to re-gain the weight—or even more weight—is not unique to the fitness world. So many times on television you see food systems being advertised that promise their diet is the best; their diet is the miraculous one that works; their diet is without doubt the best one out there, because it's been proven by science. Then, when people are no longer on those diets, they re-gain the lost weight, and then some. Don't be fooled by anyone or anything that promotes weight loss by removing entire food groups from your life.

Let's summarize the entire situation in a few sentences, and you be the judge as far as determining whether the word "health" has anything to do with any of what I just said. You basically eat a bunch of crap with the justification that you are putting on solid muscle only to later spend the other half of the year starving your body to the point of malnutrition so you look like a rock star according to industry standards. Meanwhile, you promote to others that the journey is a healthy and wonderful one to gain followers who will ask for advice on how to lose weight. When that's done, repeat again next year. Ladies and gentlemen, that was my life for almost six years.

I had a mask on that made me feel and look invincible, but I was far from those things. I was an extremist, but even then, my own judgment wouldn't allow me to harm myself that much. That, my friends, is the reality most competitors and a lot of fitness models face. There will be those who criticize me for writing this, but deep down they know it's true—and sad. If you feel your life is slightly unbalanced, it doesn't mean you have an addiction; it simply means that you should evaluate on a daily basis where most of your actions are headed. Doing so can be weird, but if you were to stop and think about your thoughts daily, you would realize there's a pattern you follow. That pattern can be modified to improve or lower your quality of life.

My personal addiction was a bundle of daily patterns that led to a choice I made to starve myself, both my body and mind. If you feel your decisions are leading to you gain weight and causing you to not make the best choices in terms of your lifestyle, then you know you need to re-evaluate things. Start there, and then brainstorm what you spend most of your time doing and thinking about on a daily basis. You, too, will start seeing your patterns. These patterns create your habits, and the habits control your actions.

- There is no such thing as a small addiction. All addictions lead to an unbalanced lifestyle that can deprive you of a healthy body and a healthy mindset. If you know you shouldn't be doing something, and yet you do it constantly, then start evaluating how you can slowly tone it down.
- Listen to what others might say about you, especially your family and loved ones. Sometimes our own egos won't allow our ears and minds to be open to suggestions that might help us.
- Don't believe there is a magic, special diet for you out there. Believe, instead, that with better eating and exercise choices, you will lose—and keep—the weight off.
- Your patterns create or destroy you. Identify the patterns you know aren't helping you, and research ways to help you slowly eliminate them from your life.

CHAPTER 5

THE CURRENT WORLD

He that takes medicine and neglects diet,
wastes the time of his doctor.
—Ancient Chinese Proverb

The sad truth is that levels of obesity—globally—keep rising. We already know this fact, yet nothing changes. Things just keep getting worse. You might wonder how this is possible, considering the vast amount of cost-effective gyms popping up everywhere, free information online, various apps, and the high number of fitness professionals out there willing to help. It all means nothing if an interest in one's health isn't valued. Do we value our health *before* some physical ailment or issue happens? No. On several occasions I've talked with many who only go to their doctor when something bothers them. Instead of taking preventative measures, the tendency is to only think of health when it's potentially too late—and when it's too late, we seek out the fast and easy way to fix things.

We never want to have to work at the long-lasting—but tedious

—solution. It's similar with our eating habits: buying fast food is fast and easy. You don't even have to walk into a restaurant anymore; just stay in the car and order, or open up an app. The only effort required is actually going to and perhaps walking from the car—and eating is eliminated. But anything that is fast and easy comes at a high price. That's right! It usually does not have a happy ending. Fast food is also cheap. But so is buying chicken, rice, and many other items in bulk. The only problem is that chicken and vegetables don't taste as good as fast food. They need to be cooked, and the entire process of getting out of your car, going into the grocery store, and then having to cook seems too long.

Does this remind you of anything else? How about going to the gym and putting in the necessary work. We live in a fast-paced society. It's all about the *now*—not later—but now. With this concept also comes the need for immediate satisfaction and reward. We want to feel good *now*, so if we're hungry, then we have to find a fast and easy way to satisfy that need. Were you actually hungry? Who knows. But you feel upset, sad, angry, in pain, etc., and you comfort yourself with food. I guarantee you that if people had to go hunt for food like our ancestors had to, or if people routinely had a twenty-minute walk to obtain food, then they'd think twice about whether they're actually hungry. But no—with two clicks on their phone and a few minutes' wait, food is there. I've done this myself after a long day of training clients. I'm no saint, but I don't do fast food on a daily basis, and the key is moderation.

We create excuses as to why things seem harder than they should be, and these daily habits slowly start to become a routine that our subconscious accepts, and doesn't want to easily change. If it literally took you a few clicks on your phone to get what you wanted, then why increase the amount of effort that's required to physically go somewhere? Make better food choices. Physical movement is eliminated daily from several things. If you've ever watched

Disney's *WALL-E*, you'll understand exactly where I'm going with this point.

People use those motorized scooters at supermarkets when they can clearly walk. Handicapped spots are given to obese people. You see the pattern. Unfortunately this is a global issue. Everywhere in the world people are slowly becoming more satisfied with going into fast food chains, eating out, and forgetting about their culinary cultures. This is not only affecting the health of individuals, but the country's traditions as well. Here's an interesting, fun fact that I learned while I was writing this book: Did you know the majority of the world's healthiest countries are in Northern Europe?

Having been raised in Europe for a large portion of my life, this makes sense. People still carry on the tradition of eating as a family, cooking as a family, and enjoying meals—they don't rush them. Ingredients are still collected from local farms, and no artificial ingredients are added to preserve shelf life since the ingredient will be cooked that same day or within the week. Cooking and passing down generations of culinary tradition is still common in Europe. For this major reason, the percentage of healthy communities is much higher. Could we learn something from them? Absolutely!

If something is three blocks away, they walk. They don't order an Uber. Daily physical movement is still a common practice, young children still walk to school, and many adults ride their bikes to work during the warm months. The increase in global obesity isn't a random occurrence. It's due to the improvement of technology (amongst other things), and the constant marketing to "improve lives." If they truly wanted to improve lives, they'd eliminate the need to find alternatives to walking, and the need for us to have to take pills to solve problems we could have already solved through exercise and eating correctly. It's hard for me to even say that statement, because I love gadgets. Trust me, I've always loved having the latest and greatest gadgets on the market, but I wouldn't buy a pair of shoes that would take away my ability to walk or download an app that took away the process of going to a restaurant, sitting down with friends, and socializing.

When I was twenty-six, I was affiliated and sponsored by a company that prepped food for athletes and for anyone who wanted healthy meals on the go. One day, the owner of the company reached out and asked me if I could help him with a small project. He wanted to go to a few underprivileged schools and educate the children about making smarter food choices. These children would more often than not get in trouble with the law or with their parents, would run away from home, and usually lacked respect for the law and their elders. I thought his idea was phenomenal, and agreed to give a speech to these young teens. The speech went extremely well, and they had a great amount of questions to ask me after I was done talking to them.

After I'd finished my presentation, one parent in attendance didn't find my speech too great. In fact, she was upset as she came over and asked me why I had told the children they shouldn't buy certain types of foods. As she was one of the parents, I had to be extremely respectful with my answer—but I also had to get a point across to her. She needed to understand that she was a role model in her house, and that providing low-quality, high-fat, high-sugar meals every day would cause her children to have future health problems. She understood my answer, and even apologized for her previous attitude. Following that, I spent an additional thirty minutes trying to educate her on food she could buy for her family that was cheap, healthy, and just took a few minutes to prepare.

Most people think eating healthy is expensive. Sure, if you go to an all-organic, natural supermarket, then prices can really be high. If you know what to buy and how to season it, though, then you can still enjoy great meals that taste amazing and are also good for you and your family. It's just a matter of learning a little about food preparation. Cooking is a skill most people don't want to learn these days. It takes time. At the end of the day, you have to ask yourself a simple question: Do I want to be healthy and learn how to be healthy? Or do I simply want the illusion of being healthy, putting forth minimal effort?

The illusion of being healthy might feed the mind for a few years, but your body will eventually speak for itself, and you'll find yourself visiting the doctor quite often. Just remember, when the medical bills start to pile up later in life and you are stressing out about money, was that cheap fast food worth the cost?

What if, when you meet a trainer and speak to them about your goals, they told you that you could lose twenty pounds or more in just a month? In return, however, you'd have to be unhealthy, lethargic, and somewhat unhappy throughout the entire process. Would you accept that offer? Would you sacrifice your health to lose those twenty pounds? I conducted my own experiment, as I was extremely curious to know what others thought about this. I personally went and asked many of my personal clients, friends, and people I randomly met at the gym what they thought of that scenario. I made sure to interview fifty women and fifty men, all between the ages of twenty-four and forty-five. This was no major scientific study, but I wanted to know for myself what choice most people would make, and why.

Here's what I obtained from my study: Women in general would not sacrifice their health for the weight. Men would. The younger ages would also make the sacrifice, but on average the people closer to their forties would not. So why was it that most younger men said they would be okay with sacrificing their health and energy levels to lose that weight, but the older demographic—and the women in general—would not? It's simple. Health is a much-more-valued component of life to those who already have families, don't care too much about how they look versus how they feel, and who, most importantly, understand the value of living a longer life.

From my experience, most people over forty understand and value the time they have on earth. They don't care about silly things like looking good to please others. What about the statistics as far as men versus women in the study? Why would more men than women choose to make the sacrifice? When I asked all fifty women why they wouldn't sacrifice their health over losing those twenty pounds, the common theme to their answers was that they better understood the fact that looks fade. A large percentage of the women—surprisingly, those on the younger end of the spectrum—even told me that having a family was much more important to them than losing weight, and if they weren't healthy enough to conceive a baby, then what was the purpose of losing weight and potentially affecting their health?

Time is the only currency we don't get back. We can't undo our mistakes, but we can use the time we currently have wisely. Nowadays we want things fast, and we don't want to waste time. Certain things, though, deserve the time to cultivate. Your health is one of them. Remember the eight-minute abs fad? If you don't know what I'm talking about, that's fine, but I'm sure you've seen an eight-week transformation challenge or a ninety-day challenge. Hell, I even offer a ninety-day challenge on my own website for those who want to work with me for three consecutive months.

Everywhere we look now, whether it's on social media or elsewhere online, we see some sort of challenge that promises to change our lives in just a few weeks. This has become such a popular trend that television networks picked up on it and created shows based around weight-loss competitions. What we don't see after those shows are over is how many of the contestants go back to their old selves, and regain the weight as fast as they lost it. We only see what they want us to see, and we believe in everything that's being told to us about the amazing results these people have obtained. They also fast-forward time, and a year-long time lapse is shown in one hour.

Some shows have gone as far as making the contestants (and us) believe that their lives are amazing now that they've lost weight, that they have no more problems. I'll say this next statement only once (so you might want to read it slowly or highlight it). Habits can't be forced out of your system. You need to re-wire your brain to rewire your life. The decisions you make now are what will sustain negative or positive habits in your life. Anyone trying to sell you on something that will change you fast and without effort is trash. In fact, my clients know from day one that the moment they start working with me, their habits are what need to start changing. No trainer is a miracle worker. The miracle worker is *you*. You are the one with all the power you need to make any changes you require. A trainer is there to teach you what you should do, to make sure you don't hurt yourself, and to sometimes hold you accountable when you don't want to show up for a hard workout.

Once again, though, a trainer shouldn't promise you that you'll be a totally different person in ninety days. Television might promote that, but as we know, what we see and watch on television or read on the internet isn't always real. It's the illusion of real. Of course, during those ninety days you can increase your strength, build lean muscle, gain power, and even lose body fat, but if you want to maintain your results and make further progress, I highly recommend you start *slowly* changing your habits so that you create a sustainable transformation. I truly dislike how the fitness industry has become an industry that promises you so much, yet most get so little. The solution to that equation is complicated, and again, it depends on you for the total sum to work.

What I do enjoy watching is those stories on social media about individuals who have dramatically changed their lives after a few years. You might read the word "years" and start to feel unmotivated—but you shouldn't. If you make changes to who you are within three years, and you get to live another fifteen to twenty years because of those three years, wouldn't you do it? If you knew for a fact that those three years of struggle and hardship would create a version of yourself you had never imagined before, why wouldn't you? Again, time is the only thing we lose in life that we can't gain back—unless that time is spent taking care of ourselves.

If you want to do a twelve-week transformation challenge, by all means, do it! But don't believe that it will only take twelve weeks to become an entirely new you. It's only the first phase or step into a potential new you. If you lose twenty pounds in those twelve weeks but were hoping to lose more, then you need to stop and realize that losing twenty pounds is better than losing no weight at all; that you took the initiative to move forward, and not remain stuck in that pondering phase.

I've seen a lot of these types of challenges, and sometimes they're more unhealthy than they are anything else. Sometimes they are created for a specific group of people only, and sometimes they're created by a person who isn't even qualified to be giving advice about nutrition or training. Additionally, these challenges can sometimes have extremely low-calorie diets with very harsh cardio requirements. Do some research on who you hire, who you want as your trainer or coach, and who you are going to seek help from. Just because the person has a huge following on social media does not necessarily make them a good choice for you. Ask questions!

People need to ask more questions, be more curious about something they're going to potentially spend a few hundred dollars on. You are investing in your health. Make the wisest choices possible. But remember, that $9.99 program could be just as good as the one that costs a thousand dollars. You are the one who will be applying the information and putting it into action, and whether the program is cheap or expensive, it won't do the work for you.

The most important thing is to never give up. If you hit a small roadblock with your trainer, your program, or life itself, just tell yourself it's a speedbump—not a wall that won't allow you to move forward. You can always move forward.

- Don't wait to reach the point of poor health, fatigue, obesity, pain, discomfort, etc. Take preventative measures today so that you don't spend thousands of dollars later as a last resort to fix something that could have been completely avoided.
- Next time you are hungry, stop and think for a second. Are you truly hungry or are you just bored? Thirsty? Or are you simply craving something to chew? Understanding how your emotions affect your eating patterns can dramatically change your views about food.
- Start thinking of all the things you currently do that allow you to eliminate the need to walk, move, or talk to someone physically in person. Start re-introducing these actions in your life.
- There's no magic to losing weight or improving your health. The magic comes from your determination, and how bad you truly want it.
- To create a sustainable transformation, don't forget about molding your mind and your habits. Doing so will ensure a long-lasting, healthier lifestyle.

CHAPTER 6

ILLUSION OF HAPPINESS

*To enjoy good health, to bring true happiness to one's family,
to bring peace to all, one must first discipline and control one's
own mind. If a man can control his mind, he can find the way
to enlightenment, and all wisdom and virtue will naturally
come to him.*

—Buddha

Happiness is a state of mind. At any given moment, you may lose it, and it may be hard to get it back. However, you have full control of that state of mind, and full control over how to gain it back. Your emotions may control almost all aspects of your daily living. Just knowing that is half the battle. A simple happy memory, thought, song, the weather, and so many other unique factors create an environment for you to be happy—but you must choose to be happy. Choosing to be happy isn't as easy as it sounds; otherwise, everyone would be walking around with a smile and problems in general wouldn't feel stressful.

For years I've been trying to find the key to success, the key to happiness, and the key to the ultimate life. I struggle with it like any other human being; some days I allow certain things that were said or done to me affect me more than usual, and on some days it's like nothing happened. But I allow that to happen to me. What does it mean to *allow* it? It means that only you have the key to the door of your mind. If you open that door and allow these emotions and feelings to enter, then you've lost control of the key, and losing that key is not good.

As I mentioned, however, you still have full control at any time, and just like training the muscles to get bigger and stronger, one must train one's mind to do the same, and prevent third party factors from affecting that state of mind. The environment we create in our minds is crucial to all of this. Your surroundings can dramatically affect the way you perceive things, and allowing people or situations to affect you can easily take away your happy state of mind. For years, my surroundings were not supporting my well-being and happiness. I was in a never-ending battle with my self-image, as it was what I believed I had to constantly work on if I wanted to be happier. My state of mind would constantly change if there was a reflection of me, and I was then reminded of my flaws.

When I discuss the illusion of happiness in this chapter, I'm talking about the perception of reality you can acquire as a result of thinking about a life you don't currently have. We all think of lives we wish we had. I'm here to help you with the health aspect of that. After all, you could be the most successful and wealthy individual on the planet, and without a healthy lifestyle, you still won't enjoy the one life that's been given to you. What I want from you after you've read this book is for you to feel and know that you have the absolute control to change what you need to change; that you don't have to look a certain way, but *feel* a certain way, in order to truly fit in and master anything you want. It is a must that you are aware that you want and need a change; otherwise, like I was in my past, you won't feel the need to change because you're living an illusion.

Does the thought of the "perfect" body bring you happiness? If it does, then you have to ask yourself why. I doubt you thought about perfect health before. If you had to choose between living until the age of seventy, having had the body of your dreams for the majority of your life, or living past your nineties, but not having the body of your dreams, which one would you choose? Unfortunately, when I asked this exact same question to so many people, the answer was they would die at seventy and have their dream body. Shouldn't the thought of living longer, with the least amount of health problems possible, bring more happiness? We tend to think only of the now, and not the tomorrow, when it comes to long-term choices. We want instant gratitude without doing any type of work.

What is it, though, that gives you the impression that having the perfect physique will improve your lifestyle? Is it because you think you would attract your soulmate? So now we're talking about love, an emotion so strong that people will do just about anything to have it. Sex sells; there's simply no doubt about that. I remember posting a shirtless picture of myself and getting four times the amount of comments and likes than I'd received with any of the purposeful posts intended to help people. Most social media pages these days that are related to fitness basically consist of women in tights showing a lot of skin. When that become a fitness trend, I don't know, but it gives the illusion that that's how women are supposed to be—and what women *should* be in order to feel attractive, healthy, successful, and happy.

What about a better house and better friends? Do you believe that the body of your dreams would attract those things in your life? A majority of the world lives under this impression, too. So did I for several years. The illusion that happiness will be obtained through being better looking is common. After all, when have you seen anyone unhappy in a commercial or ad who was sexy and skinny? You don't. You don't see the average person on any type of commercial, ad, or movie. Why? Because we don't want to see average. We want to see and imagine ourselves at the feet of the pretty and sexy people. Isn't this the same as the idea that money brings happiness, that money will solve all our problems? It's the magic thing that will also attract new friends, and bring you a new loved one.

Let me tell you, after years of training some of the richest people in Colorado, money definitely did not bring these individuals any happiness. They actually had as many—or more—problems than most people who made not even a fraction of the money these people made. Same with looks. I know hundreds of female models who are outstandingly, drop-dead gorgeous, and they complain about the same problems overweight people do. You see, that dream body isn't what's going to fix your problems. It's *you* and the power of your mindset that will. It's how you perceive the world around you and how you respond to it.

Here's a concept you should think about. The very wealthy clients I trained worked hard for their wealth and success, but like most, they thought that if the perfect body was added to their list of accomplishments, it would make their lives better. See the pattern? The people who don't have as much wealth want to achieve their dream body because they believe it will attract money and happiness. The people who have abundant wealth also believe their dream body will attract happiness, and more. One group wants what the other has, yet neither group is happy and both believe the one thing they mutually can't have without work will make their lives better. Illusions are things we believe to be true, yet are not real. It's always the things we don't have that we want.

The illusion of happiness comes in so many different forms: money, health, materialistic possessions, etc. Yet true happiness isn't from the things we think we need, but from appreciation for the things we currently have, and the things we can do to help others. I am not going to lie. I struggle with appreciating the things I have today. I had an amazing childhood with loving parents, I live in an extremely nice area of Denver, I drive a luxury car, I have an amazing woman in my life, and I have food on my table every day. Yet I still do not appreciate the things I have, and I keep focusing on the things I want. It's a complicated concept to grasp, and daily we take things for granted. That's unfortunately the norm these days.

New electronic gadgets come out monthly, new fancy clothes daily, and we want the latest and greatest. But how about your health? Why don't we want to upgrade our health daily to its version of the latest and greatest? After all, your body is the one materialistic thing that will run, and will only upgrade itself with the work *you do*. You cannot buy it; you have to earn it. I can't describe to you how amazing a good workout feels once you've learned to appreciate what it does for you. By taking the necessary daily steps, you too can upgrade your mind daily to improve upon your habits so that you always run on the latest software for your life. Exercise and eating well result in a euphoric feeling that no one will be able to give you. You need to seek it for yourself, and work on yourself daily.

When you've traveled the world like I have, a better sense of appreciation starts occurring. You start seeing how third-world countries work, and how people survive. When was the last time you had to survive to do anything? People might complain constantly that the United States is going downhill, that the current president is the worst of all time, that the economy isn't good, that racism is sky-high, etc., but these aren't people who are happy to be alive. They aren't having to survive to live. They just *live*, and take things for granted. Most of these people are the ones who would prefer to die earlier on in life with more materialistic possessions than they would prefer to live longer and truly enjoy life for what it is, creating memories that you will never forget.

The crisis in Venezuela or the Aleppo situation in Syria are constantly being shown on TV, but what immediately follows the news is a new truck commercial, and you start wishing you had the means to buy it. You've created an illusion of disappointment in your life that can never be filled. Never truly appreciating the things you currently have will always lead to wanting more and more. You need to enjoy your present and allow the future to unveil itself, but take current action today to ensure that tomorrow will be better. This means taking care of your health and body today so that tomorrow you aren't still daydreaming of what you don't have. Creating a state of happiness you can maintain means taking care of your mind, body, and soul.

Exercise has been shown in countless studies to make people happier and live longer. For once, do something out of your comfort zone. Not just for you, but for those around you, too. If you are upset and depressed that you are overweight, then change that state of mind by exercising and thinking about how it could perhaps affect your loved ones. Inspire those around you by taking action and dropping the food you know isn't helping you stay on track. One of the hardest things I've learned as a trainer is how to motivate others to change their state of mind. I can change their minds during that one hour we train, but for the other twenty-three hours they are in control. Not me.

Everyone lives a different life, and I can't commit to being a hotline my clients can text or call whenever life gets hard and they need to vent. I can, however, commit to making everyone understand that life isn't meant to be easy, that life isn't meant to be perfect, and that you only get one. If you want to go out and eat everything in sight, drink, and not exercise, then so be it, but you will be paying the consequences in this lifetime. Why choose to create short-term pleasures and live with long-term problems when you can take immediate action and live a life of balance? Balance to enjoy life in its fullest sense.

Let me share a story. Let's call this particular client of mine Barry. When I met Barry I immediately thought he was around his late thirties. He came to me asking for help, as he wanted to drop weight. Barry was one of these Instagram sensations who had close to a million followers. When I took a quick glance at Barry's Instagram page, I noticed all he did was party in fancy boats, go to clubs, and drink a lot. He had the means to do it, too. I asked Barry what made him seek my help, and he said that he didn't want to get to the age of thirty and be out of shape anymore. He also mentioned that at his last doctor's visit, his blood work hadn't been good.

I was shocked to learn that Barry wasn't even thirty years old, but it made sense after looking at all of his Instagram posts more carefully. His life seemed amazing on Instagram. Surrounded by women, money, and the glamorous life most people only dream of. I could feel and sense that Barry was actually concerned to some extent about reaching his mid-thirties and really having medical problems due to his current life choices. I was glad he sought help, as doing so can be one of the hardest things anyone can do. I was at least happy that Barry knew by that point that he wasn't indestructible, by any means.

We worked together for a few months, and it was hard to motivate him. I kept telling him that he had to slow down on the parties and drinking if he wanted to better himself. One day we spoke for a while after our session, and he opened up. He mentioned that it was hard for him to slow down with that lifestyle because he loved the attention he got on social media from the posts he created and the feeling of having so many people around him who were having a good time. I was a bit in shock that he cared so much about how others saw him, both online and in real life, that he would be willing to sacrifice his health along the way. I had done something similar with my own life when I competed.

I tried teaching him the meaning of balance, but it was tough for him to understand. I also tried teaching him the meaning of being truly happy with everything he had, but he wanted more. Barry and I trained for about a year until he moved from Colorado. I only heard of him again years later when a mutual friend told me Barry had been in the hospital for a few days due to kidney problems. Seemed things had not changed at all. In my life, I try to help as many people as possible, but they must want to open up and receive that help. After they are ready to change their mindsets and are willing to accept help, they must work in their own time to better themselves, creating the habits necessary to not only achieve happiness, but also sustain it. Remember, it doesn't have to be an illusion. You can actually create a sustainable life if you believe you can. Once you believe, and you know you are ready for change, then nothing can stop you.

You've heard me say it before, but in order to change your world, your circumstances, and your health, you must first change your mindset. It can be one of the most challenging things to truly master, but only when you start working on this will you start seeing the changes you've been wanting in your life. Later in chapter nine, you'll learn about the connection between mind, body, and soul, but for now, I want you to understand that if you don't change how you see yourself at this instant—and I mean *right now*—then it doesn't matter whether you lose a hundred pounds or gain twenty pounds of lean muscle in the next year. You will constantly keep seeing the person you were on day one.

Many feel that if they had the perfect body, they would magically gather this ultimate self-esteem that would change everything. If you can't master confidence being overweight or underweight, don't think that having the ideal body will change that. Once shy, always shy—unless you change it immediately. When I was around twenty-five or twenty-six, I had a guy come up to me while I was training and ask if I would take a picture with him. Happily, I put my weights down and stopped to take the picture with him. Soon after, he said, "Man, I wish I could look like you and go out to pick up all the girls at the clubs." I just smiled and didn't reply.

Honestly, I didn't have anything to say, because that's not the type of person I am. After he left, I didn't put too much thought into what he'd said, since I was in the middle of my training and I wanted to keep my focus on that. As I thought about it later while driving back home, though, I started remembering people telling me similar things. The same type of remarks, how if they looked like me they'd take advantage of the circumstances and go out to meet people to hook up with. I knew at the age of seventeen when I started working out that it was definitely cool when the ladies took a second look at me because of my body. But at the age of twenty-five or twenty-six, all of that was completely gone, and fitness was a means of living for me. Not a way to meet women.

Meeting random strangers was never my thing. I needed to meet people with common interests. That's why in college I was honestly not a ladies' man. Not only did I barely go out, but when I did, seeing women drinking and puking their brains out wasn't appealing to me. Knowing how to be confident will get you further than will having a bigger chest. But let's keep moving on. Whether you want to believe me or not, I'm going to tell you something personal. I have never seen myself the way others see me. I've never thought of myself as better looking or more deserving of anything because of my looks. People come in different shapes, sizes, skins, and more. To judge others because they weren't in shape was something I did during the worst years of my life. Later on I learned I had become something I hated, and I opened my eyes for the first time.

I'm telling you right now, whether you lose five pounds or a hundred, if you can't change the way you feel and the way you think about yourself, you won't be able to truly change as you expect. Sure, the outside looks better, but the inside still needs work. This illusion of happiness that you create with the anticipation of a better body changing everything about your life won't happen if you don't first create an image of who you want to be on the *inside*.

This was the case with one of my girlfriend's clients. She was about eighty pounds overweight and her goal was to lose all of it. I had trained her a few times that prior year. She worked with my girlfriend for about a year, and the weight came off. I hadn't seen her that much, as my schedule and my girlfriend's didn't match up that often, so I didn't know how she looked after dropping that weight. One day I was asked to train her because my girlfriend's schedule was too busy that day. When the woman walked into the studio, she looked like a completely different person. If I had seen her in a public place I probably wouldn't have recognized her. She looked like one of those contestants from an extreme makeover show you see on TV. I mean, a *whole new person* on the outside, with a new wardrobe, hairstyle, etc. If I hadn't known who she was from having previously met her, I would never have guessed she'd been eighty pounds overweight.

As we warmed up, I couldn't stop flattering her with compliments, and was truly excited for her. Shockingly—and sadly—she wasn't happy with the eighty pounds she had lost. She had even lost an additional ten pounds beyond her goal. She spoke to me like the ninety pounds wasn't enough, and I could hear in the tone of her voice how insecure she still was about herself. She sounded exactly like herself a year before, before any of the changes she had worked so hard to make, criticizing herself for not doing a better job. I had to immediately stop her and get her off the treadmill so we could have a talk. I knew exactly what was going on.

During the year she had lost weight, she was basically alone for most of the time, and interacted with others rarely. She worked from home, so she had no coworkers to congratulate her on the amazing job she'd done. No loved ones either, so there was no one around to truly make her feel good about her changes. I was in shock that someone who had changed so much had only managed to change the outside. I re-enforced to her that even though she'd made some amazing changes and had changed her habits, that still wasn't enough. Sometimes we don't realize how much we have changed until we stop and think about it.

When was the last time you did that for yourself? Without things turning into a therapy session, I kept training her that hour, asking her questions about her transformation. I'm not going to lie, I was super fascinated by the changes she'd made without even realizing she'd made them. She kept telling me that changing her habits hadn't been too hard. There was really no one apart from herself to sabotage her. That right there was incredible—that she realized she was her own worst enemy—but once again, she didn't give herself any credit for it. We are our own worst enemies all the time.

Since she had to lose the weight due to medical conditions, she knew she *had* to do it; there was no way around it. I asked her if she had any pictures from when she began losing the weight, and she said she didn't. I wanted to see if she could simply sit down, look at herself in the mirror, and then look at the pictures; if that would help her to realize the change. Afterwards, however, I realized that wouldn't have helped, because she saw something different than what we all did. She didn't like being in pictures, which made sense. The only way I could relate to her was by explaining that I, too, sometimes saw the 145-pound version of myself in the mirror, but I had to force myself to stop believing it.

Seeing is believing, so if you see something in the mirror that isn't there, how are you supposed to know what to believe in? It takes time, and I told her the best way to break that habit was to read books on confidence-building, and to force herself to destroy her limiting beliefs. The hard part was that she had already destroyed so many of her own limiting beliefs and hadn't realized her achievement. The same way I knew she worked her butt off to lose weight, I knew she could work her mind into slowly seeing something new that would change her life and bring her potential happiness and peace. That's why the balance of health cannot solely come from your physical body; it has to be an equal balance of mind, body, and soul for you to truly succeed.

The last bit of advice I gave her was about how I struggle with myself, but in a financial aspect. If you are going to measure success and happiness based on numbers, then you will constantly struggle to achieve what you seek, and you'll be disappointed. Numbers are infinite, so trying to see the numbers on the scale as they drop in order to seek happiness will create a never-ending battle with yourself. Don't allow the illusion to become your reality.

- Control your state of mind with music, videos, funny moments, and positive memories. At any given moment you can turn your emotions around and control them to your advantage.
- Wanting something and needing something are two different things. Most people just want something, but if they really needed that something, they would do what it takes to get it. Next time you set a goal, start by telling yourself "I need to . . . " instead of saying "I want this or that." One is wishful thinking, the other is goal-setting.
- The perfect body will not bring you happiness, money, friends, or a better life. Your state of mind will, and you can start working on that immediately.

- Ask yourself this: Do you have a roof to shelter you daily? Food available at any given moment you desire it? Clothes to keep you warm? If so, then you are already at more of an advantage than many in the world. The only reason you can't see it is because you take having these life essentials for granted. Take a minute daily to be thankful for what you already have earned and achieved in this lifetime.
- Asking for help can be one of the hardest things to do, yet once you know that change must happen, seek help from those who are experienced. Then, take action daily.

CHAPTER 7

BEING TOO HEALTHY: IT'S UNHEALTHY

*Everyone has their own definition of a healthy lifestyle,
and mine has come to mean making health a priority
but not an obsession.*

—Daphne Oz

How is it possible for someone to be so healthy that it becomes unhealthy? Technically it's not. For years I was under the impression that I was a healthy individual, yet I was constantly getting sick throughout the year, I was stressed and anxious, and my mind wouldn't see food. It would see numbers. The perspective I had of my own wellness was an illusion. It's no surprise that when you focus only on one area of your wellness that the others fall short. This applies to any circumstance in your life as well, not just your health. I believed that focusing on every single aspect of the food I ate was key, and because of it I developed orthorexia along the way. What is orthorexia? It's an obsession with defining and maintaining the perfect diet. It makes you fixate on eating certain foods, but you might fear an entire food group.

In my case, it was carbs and sugars. Carbs were the enemy, as traditional bodybuilding diets and athletes always said that in order to get to a body-fat percentage in the single digits, you'd have to eliminate as many carbs as possible. After I was done with a show, though, I would stuff my face with as many carbs as possible, and feel my body hating me for days. You stop enjoying the food itself and start treating it like a mandatory requirement based on its nutritional content and value. Normally, no one looks at a banana and has this train of thought: "It's roughly twenty to twenty-five grams of carbs, but let's make sure by weighing it down to truly see how many grams it is. Plus, the banana will have a fast insulin spike, so I should only consume it before and after a workout, and if I eat this at night I will gain fat." Now imagine this process with all the foods you eat in a day. You go crazy!

I went to the extreme, but isn't that what's going on in the media as well? Isn't this what you see on TV and read in magazines about your favorite celebrity? That the celebrity had a "new, special diet" that was low in fats, carbs, gluten, sugars, etc.? And after you read their stories and see their pictures, you think to yourself, "This is the diet I should be on!" You might lose a few pounds at first, but then hit a wall. Then you read about a whole new diet someone else did, and once again, you say, "Now this is the diet for me. The other one simply wasn't for me." Unless you change your lifestyle to a path of better decision-making, none of these diets will ever fit your lifestyle—because your lifestyle for the past however many years had *nothing to do with taking care of your health.*

You can't force yourself into a new lifestyle that easily. For me, it was a lifestyle, but an extreme one, where I wouldn't allow myself to eat anything unless it has a purpose behind it. Trainers, nutritionists, and media out there always tell us to keep an eye out as far as what we eat, what we consume in the late hours, and what we drink daily. But take this to the next level and you don't see food anymore.

You see numbers. I remember back in my competing phase, a coworker once asked me if I enjoyed eating tilapia and veggies for almost all of my meals for multiple weeks. I clearly remember my answer. I told her that food was just food; it was just macros, and not intended for taste, basically just solid matter for existence. It was there to provide me with energy and recovery. That's it. I'm never going to forget her expression; it was if she was looking at an alien.

I can look back now and only laugh. Our bodies have taste buds for a reason, and I clearly I did not understand that at the time. Did I enjoy eating the same thing over and over again? Absolutely not, but it was what I needed to do in order to win, or at least look my best to place higher. Winning meant everything to me. There was no second place in my mind, so I would do whatever it took to earn that spot. At the 2016 Mr. Olympia Weekend I was catching up with a friend who was still competing. She had been competing for about fifteen years, and when I told her I was done with the lifestyle it almost seemed like she was upset at me. "How can you stop, Alex?! You were one of the original founders of the division you competed in!"

In my mind, that didn't mean anything to me anymore, as I had found balance and a meaningful purpose for my life. As I was explaining my idea for this book to her, she actually got upset when I described food as more than just a number or macro. She honestly did not like it that I told her she needed to take a break from that lifestyle in order to see what life is truly about. I was the exact the same way if anyone talked to me about food, but now I was on the other side and could see how ridiculous it was. What's sad is that this wasn't just one case. There were thousands of individuals I knew who still thought of food, and life in general, in those terms.

Unfortunately, another habit I developed was the over-consumption of vitamins and supplements. I feel like self-medication is common these days. For instance, do you have a head ache? Pop a pill. Have a minor ache in your neck? Pop another pain pill. Pills are used like water, without even truly thinking of the adverse, long-term consequences. You are probably going to laugh when I say this, or maybe think I'm just plain nuts, but back in those days I was popping about twenty-two pills for breakfast, around fifteen throughout the day, and another twenty-two before bedtime. I needed to make sure I had all my vitamins, minerals, and dietary supplements for recovery and stamina. I was taking close to sixty pills a day!

Sure, people who train hard and are constantly exposing their bodies to harsh training conditions should have an extra boost, but I doubt that equals anywhere near sixty pills a day. I remember my habit had already begun in high school when I used to take a multi-mineral/vitamin combination of eight pills. My friends used to make jokes and say I was a junkie, but what began as eight pills, progressed to more and more over time. I remember in January 2011, I went to my physician to get a regular beginning-of-the-year checkup. On the pre-appointment sheet, this was one of the questions: "Are you taking any supplements? If so, please list them." As I filled in that sheet, I ended up not having enough space to write everything, so I continued writing on the back of the paper.

I thought it was a bit comical, but the doctor didn't. He asked me why I took so many pills and supplements a day, and I answered that my diet was a bit restrictive, that I felt like I needed to supplement the nutrients I was not obtaining naturally from food, and that the other supplements helped my recovery and provided me with energy. Food should naturally give anyone energy; however the meals I was eating at the time didn't contain too many micronutrients, so I started depending on these supplements for mental and physical energy. Basically I was under nourished, and I was pushing my body to the limits, trying to supplement my life with every possible product.

The doctor gave me the same look my coworker had, like they'd just met E.T. I didn't think there was anything out of the ordinary about it, as everyone I spoke to on a regular basis and those I talked to whenever I competed, were all doing the same or more. Thinking back, when the guys met up and discussed all the products we were taking, if someone was taking something the rest of us weren't, then we would wonder how much of an extra boost that one supplement could provide. We would all do our research and buy it later. Instead of war stories, we shared dumb-habit stories that we, in a way, felt proud of. The dumber the thing we did, the more we felt it was honorable to share. Once again, we were the models hired for health posters, ads, and commercials; we were the ones you'd see in magazines promoting healthy habits and healthy eating—it was far from that, by a long shot. The hypocrisy.

The mind is limitless; however, the body is not. When you start working out for hours a day, you start taxing your body and losing sense of what is healthy for you. You start losing sense of time and life itself; the only thing you know is the reflection in front of the mirror. If you aren't happy with it, you just keep pushing harder. That was my reality. That was the reality so many of my friends had, too. Guess what? That's called body dysmorphia, something I still battle with sometimes. A small part of you says you've had enough, while the other part says you can do more. You look at yourself in the mirror and see something that displeases you. No matter how good you look, it's not good enough, and you criticize yourself more and more.

Everyone around you might say you look perfect, but in your head you see the version of yourself that you least like. You see all your flaws, and start comparing them with people around you, or with those you follow on social media. "You're not there yet," is what I used to tell myself whenever I had mental images of the people I knew were going to be onstage with me. No matter how hard I dieted and exercised, I felt fluffy; that I did not have enough muscle. We all criticize ourselves a little on a daily basis, but what I would do is rip myself apart with the idea that doing so would push me to train harder and eat less.

We all sometimes wish we could just lose a little fat and tighten up, but body dysmorphia is much more than that. It would affect my daily mindset so much that all my actions would be based on how I saw myself—the same way as the client who'd lost ninety pounds and still wasn't pleased. I would look at myself dehydrated, at 4 percent or less body fat, and find flaws to work on. It took me a few years after ending my competing phase to piece back together the puzzle pieces in my mind. I thought people had to look a certain way to be physically fit. They had to have a sculpted abdominal section, eighteen-inch biceps, veins coming out of everywhere, etc., but the reality is that normal human beings aren't meant to be in that type of condition. We're meant to function and be internally healthy.

I clearly remember waking up one morning and unfollowing roughly a thousand people on my Instagram feed. Took almost two hours. I was fed up seeing bodies like that. Who knew how many Photoshop edits had been done to their photos, how many takes it potentially took to get that perfect shot, or how tan and dehydrated the models were in order to showcase the perfect picture. I no longer wanted to see any of that, as I knew I had a problem, and I wanted to compare myself. The next day I decided to start following people in the wellness community: yoga instructors, companies that promoted healthy living, physically and mentally. I still follow close friends who compete, but the majority of people who impact me on any type of social media platform are those sharing happiness and wellbeing. Who are you following on social media? Why? How do they inspire you to live a healthier life and how to do they make you feel?

The problem didn't stop with just taking too many pills, seeing food as numbers, and my body dysmorphia. Oh no, I felt that all of these added up, and I slowly started developing a sense of obsessive compulsive disorder. For those who don't know what that is, I'll explain. It involves having excessive thoughts that lead to repetitive behavior compulsions. Maybe some of you saw this one coming, but I surely did not. Everything in my life had a daily pattern, and had to be absolutely perfect and consistent in the way I did it. I felt the need to arrange my food in specific ways. Carbs had to stay on one side, proteins and fats on the other. Luckily, I caught on to these things faster than I did my other negative behaviors, and was able to slowly turn it around.

Can I honestly say it's all gone? Probably not. I still today need to have my things very well organized or I start getting anxious and stressed. Silly things, too, like kitchen utensils and my computer desk. How being in the gym daily for hours and calculating my food to the exact, precise amount lead to so many problems, I don't know. One thing just lead to another, until one day I realized with the help of my girlfriend that none of it was technically normal. Normality is hard to define, as each one of us has a different perspective of life, but when you can't function properly, even in your own reality, that's when you know it's no longer normal.

Personally, I don't like using the word "normal," but I knew that all those habits needed to stop if I ever wanted to be happy with myself and with anyone who would be with me. If you know you have a problem, then the first person you need to talk to is yourself. Sit down, analyze the situation, and reflect on why you believe it's happening. Trace it backwards and determine the factors that led to each phase. Only you have the power to love and cure yourself of so many of your self-perceived problems.

- Look at yourself in the mirror first thing in the morning and repeat to yourself, "I am strong, I am beautiful, and I will have an amazing day ahead." Love yourself.
- No diet is going to fit your lifestyle. You create a lifestyle to fit the new habits you will maintain to succeed and sustain a better life.
- Are the influencers you follow on social media providing you with ideas on how to be a better version of yourself? If not, why do you really follow them?

CHAPTER 8

FINDING YOUR FIT

When we stop comparing ourselves with others,
we are then free to stand in our own light.
—Linda Field

When you seek to do something different in life, don't look at what others are doing, seek within yourself and find out what makes you happy and motivated. What's your favorite clothing brand? How about your favorite color? There are so many answer options for those two questions, yet the majority of people will answer them with a generic choice. There's nothing wrong with choosing something generic, but you will soon see my point. Instead of ruby, rose, merlot, berry, mahogany, crimson, etc., which are all shades of red, most people would just say "red." "I like red." Nothing wrong if you like black, blue, red, or any standard, plain color, but those are the base colors. They are generic options without variation to them. Most people will also have chosen their favorite clothing brand based on the big-name brands you usually see when you walk into a sports store. Makes sense; the more a company can afford to put toward marketing, the more visible it usually becomes to customers.

Did you know that in California they have a yoga class based on animals? That's right, it's an entire yoga class based on poses that resemble animals. In Spain they have Bossaball, a volleyball game that's played with trampolines and foam mats. What about sex-ercise? You read that right. Sex movements performed at an exercise-level cardio rate. At first these things might sound odd, but so was for millions of people when Crossfit was first introduced and in its original form.

When most think about setting goals and wanting to exercise, they lack originality in their options, and immediately think of either running outside or joining a gym and lifting weights. In fact, running is the most common form of exercise globally. It's free, and you can do it almost anywhere you live. But what if you don't enjoy running? What if you have bad knees from previous injuries or the weather isn't in your favor? I remember I once had a client—let's call her Lucy. I'm never going to forget Lucy, as she was one of the most negative and depressed clients I had ever worked with. The first time I met her she explained to me that she wanted to lose ten pounds for her wedding that was coming up, but she also told me she didn't want to exercise in order to achieve that goal, and she did not want to diet.

I looked at Lucy and replied, "Then what do you really want with a personal trainer?" In the back of my mind I already knew Lucy would be a complicated individual to work with, but I always liked a challenge. Lucy explained that she really didn't like to exercise because she didn't like to be sore after any type of workout. Additionally, she didn't feel like dieting because she had a social life to keep up. She didn't want to give that up in order to lose the weight she told me she wanted to lose. She came to me because she'd heard from someone that I got clients great results. I explained to Lucy that the reason I had that reputation wasn't because I pushed my clients until they couldn't move the next day, it was because my clients put forth the effort to reach their goals on their own. With my help, I could be their dependability and motivation to come workout.

I also like to talk to my clients to understand their lifestyles so we can work around what they think are their challenges so exercise and proper eating could become part of their daily life. Lucy further explained that she had heard on the news that there was a new medication the FDA was going to potentially approve that would allow people to lose weight without making any changes to their current lifestyle.

I told Lucy those things did not work, and without any type of effort she wouldn't reach her goals. She wasn't too pleased with my answers, as I believe deep down she thought I had a magic potion to give her. Lucy's consultation did not end so well. She ended up getting irritated that everything I told her had some form of commitment-related aspect to it, and she didn't want to do any of that. My last suggestion was for her to try different types of classes offered at her local gym and see if any of them would be to her liking.

I didn't see Lucy for a few months, until one morning I bumped into her at a local Whole Foods and saw her buying a salad. I was a bit shocked she was eating a salad, but I was happy for her and asked her how things were going. She was actually happy to see me, which, in turn, I was too shocked about. She explained that a few days after we had met she saw an ad for a gym that trained people like circus dancers. Personally, I had never heard of this before, so I was extremely curious to hear about it. She told me this studio in Denver trained individuals to be like the sensual ballerinas you see at circus shows.

The classes consisted of a mixture of ballet, yoga, and acrobatics. Honestly, Lucy was the last person in my mind who would ever even consider—or walk into—a place like that, but she did, and she looked like she had lost her ten pounds and was more motivated than ever. The lesson of this story is that even *I* was being closed minded when I'd seen Lucy walk in and couldn't find her fit. You do have to be opened minded when trying to find your fit, as traditionally you will want to do things inside your comfort zone. It's when you do things you'd never thought of doing, that you open your life to new experience and opportunities. Take Lucy's example and do some research on different styles of exercise and classes you can take or do at home so that you can *enjoy* being healthy. Don't fall victim to what's being marketed the most. Get out of our comfort zone and try the unthinkable.

One of the most common things I hear from people when they're thinking about losing weight is how tedious the treadmill can be. I always wonder why the treadmill is the first image or machine that comes to people's minds when they think about the gym. The usual answer is because their home, apartment complex, or local gym has a lot of treadmills, and that's the easiest thing to do. Makes sense, though; all you have to do is jump on any machine these days and there's a big green button that says "Quick Start." You don't even have to set up any options to begin—no weight, no height—nothing. Just hit that button and go.

If you remember, I'm not a fan of the words "quick" or "fast." For one moment think about your local gym or any gyms you've walked into before. What's the first thing that you usually see past the front desk? Machined dedicated to cardio workouts. Rows and rows of cardio machines. They will show you the gym, and talk proudly of how much cardio equipment they have. There's a reason for that, and why all the barbells and dumbbells are in the back, farthest from the entrance. Most people feel intimidated or overwhelmed by barbells and dumbbells. Machines aren't bad, because most of them have instructions or are self-explanatory; although I must admit, I have seen some crazy things on machines that were not originally meant for the purpose they ended up creating.

Barbells and dumbbells are old school; they're heavy and they can make too much noise, which brings attention to you if you use them. They also tend to be in front of large panels of mirrors. Not only do you have to look at yourself while you exercise, but others look at you, too. For the fitness beginner or new gym member, they typically don't want that. They want something easy and fast that doesn't draw attention; something that won't make them feel uncomfortable. Look, I'm never going to judge you on what you do at the gym, but isn't the point of going there to make you feel slightly uncomfortable to begin with?

A sense of being uncomfortable means that something needs to be changed, and you have the full power to do so. Sometimes as I walk into a gym I feel like I'm watching cattle; everyone doing the same thing and on their phones. Sounds harsh to put it that way, but it's true. No wonder a large percentage of the population cannot make a positive association to exercise. You must find your fit in order to enjoy the experience. Truth is, there are days I don't want to even *think* of a gym, but I do it because I know it's good for me and for my health. I no longer use the gym as a drug to hide my emotions, my feelings, or obsessing about my body, but instead I use it as a place for physical and mental improvement.

You need to have a different outlook about something you might not enjoy in order for it to become a part of your life and help you reach your goals. We only have one body, one mind, and one soul. Our health depends on those three, and you only get one of each of those things in this lifetime. Get used to being uncomfortable at first so that you can eventually make it a routine that you proudly enjoy performing . . . so let's find your fit!

STEPS TO FINDING YOUR FIT

• • •

- What's your goal? Weight loss? To be healthier? Increase muscle mass? You need to know what you truly want. After all, you won't add pounds of muscle by attending a yoga class, or lose weight just by doing Pilates. Know exactly what you want, and be honest with yourself. Keep it simple: "I want to lose fifteen pounds"; "I want to gain five pounds of lean muscle"; "I want to be more agile and flexible."
- Be realistic with your goals. It's important to set goals; otherwise, how will you measure your success? Too many people set goals that are too high for the time period in which they desire to accomplish them. False expectations based on something you saw can lead to failure. You are unique, and your body will respond differently than other people's. Losing ten pounds in two weeks is not realistic or healthy. Losing one to three per week is. Set short- and long-term goals for yourself. One example of a short-term—and realistic—goal: "I want to lose two pounds this week, but by next month I want to have lost eight pounds total."
- Research: Most people, as I mentioned, don't research. They simply do what they already know, or what others are telling them. Go online, read books, and talk to experts. Research what ways you can get in shape and achieve your goals. If you are looking to increase your mobility and flexibility, then yoga and Pilates are great initial paths to start, but they're not the only paths available. If you are looking to be healthier, then looking at nutritional seminar to improve your knowledge on cooking and eating is a great

start, too. Do a little research beyond the first five things you see in your web browser, and examine how that activity is reviewed by others.

- Try: This is one of the most important points. Researching and not actually doing it will be a waste of your time. You must break out of your shellf and try new things. I personally did not enjoy yoga, and it was hard for me to go into a yoga studio, but I tried it several times, and I can confidently say that's it not for me.. Later I tried Pilates and loved it. Similar concepts to each other, but different with outcomes. The beauty of it is that most places will give you a free trial of their class or gym so you can see if you like it or not. You won't know until you try.

- Repeat and be consistent: Did you finally find something you like? Good! You shouldn't rush in finding what you like. After all, this will be something you'll have to repeat multiple times. Building a positive relationship with the activity or location will make you want to come back and repeat the process. Give something more than one chance. I didn't like yoga the first time, but I tried it a few more times. It simply wasn't for me. When I first tried Pilates, I enjoyed it much more than yoga. By being uncomfortable, your mind will create an environment for emotions you might not enjoy. As you slowly break that sense of feeling out of place, you'll create more positive emotion, which will boost your interest in the activity. I'm not saying do something for an entire month that you obviously know you don't like after your initial experience of it. But if you still have doubts, and can't decide if it's for you, keep giving it a try. It's just like dating. You don't know your match unless you go out and spend time with the other person to determine if you are compatible together.

- Start all over again if you must. You're probably thinking, He's crazy! I just did all this, and I have to start all over again?! You read right. Sometimes the activity we liked so much in the first three months simply gets boring. It's not challenging you anymore, or you lost interest in it; however, it served its purpose for a few months as a way to initiate your spark, and now you just need to find something else to keep you going. There's nothing wrong with that. You just need more stimulation, and switching things up or taking part in multiple types of exercise is what gets you going.

- Do it for yourself. Don't go through these steps and feel like you must do any of it if your motivation is to please someone else. You most definitely can bring a friend, or try something new with a few of your friends, but at the end of the day, whatever activity you choose must be yours to enjoy. It must be your "thing."

There you have it! Seven steps to finding your fit. Don't get disappointed if you go to a few places and don't like it. After all, you wouldn't order something from a menu at a restaurant if you didn't like it. But in order to find out whether you like something, you usually try it first. Another thing to consider when trying to finding your fit is whether you are a lone wolf or a group person. Never say no to something you haven't tried, because you might like it. Personally, I've tried group classes multiple times, and they simply aren't my cup of tea—but I can say I tried them. On the other hand, if you feel like you are motivated by others being in a group setting, and you don't do well on your own, then stick with that . . . but try slowly stepping out on your own as well. You might enjoy the one-on-one time you get with yourself.

For years, I was never the type to try different things. Today, I will try most things. Zumba and ballet might not be on that list of things to try right now, but I will never say never. I've met so many shy people over the years who felt like the gym was the last place on earth where they belonged, but after a few weeks I couldn't stop seeing them in there. They didn't just change physically over time, but they became happier socially, and became friendlier individuals, too. It's incredible to see the changes people go through when they allow change to enter their lives, and allow their barriers to come down. In fact, so many of my former clients and acquaintances actually met their significant others when they were in environments they never thought they'd personally be in—until they started taking care of their health. By exposing yourself to new places you traditionally wouldn't go to, you increase your chances of making new friends and having new experiences in your life.

- The companies that have the most money have the most marketing behind them. Don't become a zombie to marketing. Think outside of the box, and be unique in your ways of thought. Try new things and experiment with what you never thought would work for you.
- Don't fall victim to life's "Quick Start" button. Take a little time and customize your workouts to meet your needs.
- Follow the seven steps to finding your fit. They are simple, and can completely change how you approach fitness.
- Creating new memories and emotions in this life requires you to do new things. Try this silly exercise: Pretend your body got possessed by a new soul, and don't even think—just act. Go online and register for a free class of spinning or yoga, or anything you once thought you wanted to try but subconsciously talked yourself out of doing. Choose somewhere close to your home, too. If it's far away, you will create excuses not to go.

CHAPTER 9

FITTING HAPPINESS INTO YOUR LIFE

Happiness is not a goal; it is a byproduct.
—Eleanor Roosevelt

The Internet can be a blessing and a curse. It can help you and confuse you at the same time. I remember searching for some information on the subject of weight loss for individuals with adrenal fatigue—which I'd experienced before. I wanted to know more information on the subject, and how it mentally affected those who had it. Wow! I only found over a few thousand sites with information. Only a few *thousand* sites. Then it clicked: I wondered how someone who didn't have any knowledge of health, fitness, or other related subjects would find the answers they were looking for on the web. Which ones should you read? Which one do you apply?

So I decided afterwards to search "weight loss." Have you ever done a search for the term "weight loss" on Google or YouTube? It feels like a maze when you look at all that information. There are over ten thousand search results. Ten thousand! No wonder people read about and try crazy things to lose weight. There were sites that promoted extremely unhealthy methods, such as eating a thousand calories a day or less; sites that even promoted fasting for a period of a few days. It all made sense to me now, the reason people had such a hard time trying to find the answers they were looking for. On top of that, I felt like the sites that paid more for the top spots on the search engines were simply trying to sell you their crazy methodologies and supplements.

The definition of crazy is relative to each and every one of us, but to drink a tea and magically lose ten pounds or more a week while keeping your same lifestyle seems crazy to me. Words such as "fast," "easy," "sexy *now*," etc. are all used in these schemes to target those who don't know any better. Let me give you a simple piece of advice that relates to anything—not just fitness and health. You've read this here before: If the words "fast" and "easy" are included in the product description, then they're not going to help you. If it was that fast and easy, then everyone would be doing it. But these websites make you feel like you've hit the jackpot; that it's a secret only a few have stumbled upon; that you have to act now, otherwise the products they are selling might run out.

There's also the before-and-after photos that promise you the individuals used the products being advertised, and they're extremely happy with their lives now. Only now, after losing all that weight, were these individuals able to achieve "true happiness." Crazy! Basically, what all these people state is that they were in a state of depression and negativity until they bought the specific products and lost some weight. Just like magic, now they are happy. Happiness is a state of mind. Let me repeat that. Happiness is state of mind. Think of just one memory right now that brings you joy and happiness, and immerse yourself in it. Remember how it made you feel at the moment, and it will automatically change the way you feel in the present.

Whether it was the birth of your son or daughter, your wedding, a special birthday or day, or even the day you got a puppy, close your eyes and think about it for one full minute. Remember the details of that moment. Think of the smells, the actions, the music that perhaps was playing, the people involved in the scene, etc. Basically try and re-live that moment just for a minute. Stop reading now, and start again when you're done with that one special thought. Take four deep breaths; in through your nose and out through your mouth. How do you feel right now? Slightly more relaxed and happy? Great! Now try and think of repeating this every time you feel upset or stressed.

So why do most people find a moment of faith or comfort when they see those before-and-after pictures of individuals who lost weight? Because you see your face and your body in those pictures, and for an instant you believe that buying those certain products or doing a certain fast and easy diet will fix your problems. This is going to sound harsh, but here's the reality: If it took you years to get in the current shape you are in now, why would it take a fraction of the time for you to be healthy and in shape? That's not how your body works. These pictures or websites try to control your emotions so that you feel a sense of relief, relief that you finally found a product you can just pop in your mouth and your weight loss problems be gone.

That quick state of happiness that results is how they sell something to you. Go now to the bathroom. Go there, look yourself in the eyes and say, "There's nothing wrong with me. I am perfect the way I am, but I know that I can work on being better with my health." That's it! What you did there is positively encourage yourself. Secondly, make a statement of action: "I will look now into my local gym, and see what classes they offer."; "I will go to the grocery store and buy the right foods for my goals." Take action as soon as you think of what you want to change. Don't allow time to go by, as your state of mind will change. Act when your state of mind is working at its best to make you feel inspired, when it's working *with* you and not against you.

You should do this every day when you wake up, too. Wake up! Don't snooze. Take action immediately instead of allowing your brain to tell you otherwise. This can be applied to everything. Start taking control of your thoughts. Your relationships, your work, your daily life, etc. Remember, you're the one who created the habits that can lead to a poor, unhealthy life. You, and only you, can—and will—do your best to change that.

So how do you apply this to your daily life? How do we get you to repeat the positive habits that will lead to better health and a better version of yourself? It just takes action on your part. It's all about habits. If you wait for the magic moment of motivation to hit you to begin acting upon what you want, then you will be waiting for a long time. People feel like they have to get motivated or inspired before they can take action and slowly create those habits. If you do that, nothing will change. You have to take immediate action without too much thinking in order to create or initiate the first act.

It's probably a habit for you to brush your teeth in the morning and at night. If it's not, I would highly encourage you to start there. Habits create, make, and destroy us. On my own quest toward self-improvement, I would spend hours reading about habits, listening to audio tapes, and researching the mechanisms that create and can also re-wire these habits. I could spend a while talking to you about how it all works, but all you need to know are a few things. It's all about likes and dislikes. What we might sometimes perceive as our dislikes, are simply actions we haven't learned to enjoy and appreciate yet. Of course, I'm not talking about sticking your finger in an electrical outlet or putting your hand on a hot surface; subconsciously you know those actions will hurt you.

When it comes to going to the gym, eating healthy, and taking actions toward your better good, doing those things doesn't *physically* hurt you. You simply haven't created the wiring to build that habit and enjoy it because at that point exercise still seems like a lot of work with little immediate reward. Just think, we all have the option to get our butts off the couch, go to the supermarket, buy healthy ingredients and cook our lunch and dinner for the day, or open an app and order your favorite pizza or Chinese meal. One is quick, effortless ,easy, and provides fast reward. See the word "easy" in there? The other takes time and action, but in the long run, is better for you.

If you—just once—go to the grocery store, buy what you need, and cook it, you've now started the creation of a new path in your brain that says, "I am making an effort to be better." You would also see that it's not as bad as you originally thought it would be. Think of it this way, too: Creating a new path in your brain is like creating a path through a jungle that no one has ever stepped foot in before. The first time you walk from your camp to the jungle to get water, you've stepped on a few leaves. The next time you go to the same spot to obtain water, there are new leaves on the floor, along with the leaves you stepped on previously. The more you walk back and forth through that path, the more of a foundation you are developing.

Eventually, there will be a path that soon turns into a walkway to that water. If that water is now a resource, and you need it daily, then your actions eventually will create a dirt path to get there. The more you walk, the more evident it is to others and to yourself that that's the route to get to water. The more you act on something, the more habitual it becomes to you. This goes both ways, though. If you constantly buy junk food, you are creating a path toward those actions. If you cook and workout regularly, then that's the path you will most likely keep following, so long as you keep repeating it.

Stop the desire for immediate reward, because in life and in your health, that won't happen. Don't allow your negative emotions to control your actions. Simply start something, no matter how unmotivated you feel. Motivation will come from doing the right things slowly. But you must take the initial unknown road.

Action can be begin at any instant; you just really need to start moving or doing something towards your goal. Here's a technique you can utilize to help you with taking actions: I was always under the impression that it was completely wrong to live my life thinking "What if?" The "ifs" of life would only lead to unsuccessful actions. But, as always, isn't that a matter of perception, too? What do I mean by all this? Well, taking action is hard for many people. For some it's easy, like with the example I used previously about going to the grocery store and buying foods you know are better for you. That right there can be hard for so many. Now let's talk about "What if?"

What if you just pictured first picking up the car keys and getting into the car. Finally, imagine going to get the groceries and coming back. Let's just start with those mental pictures. Don't even worry about imagining cooking the food and eating it. Take it step by step. Now what if you just took a quick second to actually grab those keys and get into your car? No analyzing the circumstances, just getting up and doing it. The "what ifs" can now turn into a real scenario. Something so small is already leading toward a great potential action, and that's where it can start for you. From there on, start asking yourself, "What if I did this or that? What would be the outcome?

If you are scared, and you imagine negative scenarios, you know you need to work on projecting a more positive outlook, and that's where you begin. What if I were to just walk around the block today and get half a mile in? What would be the result of that? That said, would it make you feel slightly better if you went for a short walk today? What if the day after tomorrow you walked that same block twice? How would that make you feel, working toward your desired fitness goals? See where I am going with this? Start visualizing what it would feel like if you did indeed take these small steps to improve yourself.

You can't always control your emotions, but this quick and small technique can make you feel like you *want* to improve a scenario, and use that positivity to take initial, small actions. You can take this process and apply it to anything you want in life: relationships, work, friends, family, and your own health. The problem is that we always visualize the big picture, but not the fragments that will lead us there. We see ourselves potentially losing thirty pounds in the next six months, but we don't know where to even start.

Think to yourself, *What if I lost thirty pounds? How would that make me feel?* Secondly, break that goal, and think, instead, *What if I lost five pounds per month? How would that make me feel?* Losing five pounds is pretty good, and it's a step in the overall direction toward losing thirty pounds. The concept is to make yourself think about how the end results will make you feel, and then break down those goals into smaller segments so you can achieve them. Let's say you responded so well, you actually lost ten pounds in a month. That state of mind of self-accomplishment leads to happiness. As I previously encouraged you to do, remember that feeling. Treasure it, click the Save button in your brain, and don't forget it. Easier said than done.

But just like the habits I'm trying to teach you to create, this is one for you to add to the list of habits that will lead to successful, healthy living. Share with others how you are doing it. After all, you know what it feels like to initially not be able to even grab the car keys and hit the grocery store. Share with those who want to know how you simply asked yourself, "What if I grabbed my keys and began my journey to happiness and health right now?" Keep repeating the process. The more you keep repeating it, the more you will break those self-imposed barriers. It's okay if you take three steps forward and one step backward; you are still two steps ahead. After all, you need to understand that you are *human,* just like everyone else, and small failures here and there are okay.

That's a concept I remind my clients of daily, in case they ever fail at something. In fact, I started asking all my clients to start our sessions by sharing with me two or three things they did outside of our training hour together to help reach their goals. Whether it's walking two miles with their family or their dogs, making a smarter decision when eating out, or even something small, like listening to a five-minute motivational video. I want everyone to create a state of happiness during our sessions—*and* outside those hours—so they can work nonstop at being their best. It's all about starting small—but *starting.* As Ralph Waldo Emerson once said, "A mind stretched by a new idea never regains its original dimensions."

- Don't wait for the lightning bolt of motivation to hit you. Create it any time you need it.
- You control how you think, hence you control how happy you can be.
- Be patient with yourself. If, for years, you've not been eating well and/or not exercising, then don't expect one week of great work to fix years of mistakes.
- Learn how to walk before you run. Learn how to think. Most importantly, act small before trying to think large. This will aid you in your new actions and habits.
- It's okay if you fail a few times in your journey toward creating better habits. Fail, then learn why you failed. This will enable you to prevent the likelihood of repeating the same small mistakes.

CHAPTER 10

VIRTUAL HAPPINESS

Happiness isn't found in a small screen, it's found in the
memories we create with those around us.

—Alex Carneiro

Are you feeling happier now that you know the necessary steps to fit your fit and change your life? You no longer need to wonder how to make it happen. Speaking of happiness, I want to dedicate a shorter chapter on how your happiness and health are affected by social media and mainstream media. You've already heard me talk a little bit about social media. But let's talk about it some more. For me, social media was not a big part of my growing up. Sure, Myspace was there, but it didn't have the impact that Facebook and Instagram has on people today.

Companies spend a large chunk of money on Facebook and Instagram these days, as more people follow their favorite brands, celebrities, influencers, and other companies. I'm happy I didn't grow up with social media, as I've seen the good and bad it does to people. Sadly, in the fitness environment I believe social media has had such an impact, that now most people draw their knowledge from posts, as opposed to books and going to the library.

In general, your happiness and emotions will constantly go up and down. That's life, and if you're spending the majority of your free time scrolling through your phone, that will impact you more than you think. Remember when I talked about spending time with one of the five people to whom you're closest? Focus on *being* with them. These days, you probably spend more time on your phone on social media than you do with any of those five people in your life.

Most young men and women spend a good amount of time checking out their favorite athletes, models, and influencers on these platforms, and the damage that can do to the unmolded mind is severe. Remember at the beginning of this book, when I asked you what you think of when you think about fitness? Most people these days think of yoga pants, tight glutes, and women barely wearing anything in order to get your attention. In fact, the majority of accounts on Instagram these days that have the most followers are those with women showing the greatest amount of skin. Health and fitness or soft-core porn? If it's entertaining, then you, too, will watch, but when did entertaining become a source of credibility when it comes to advice about health?

I am not judging anyone for what they post, but I will judge how their posts affect minds in respect to what "healthy" should look or be like. I'm not okay with a guy or girl with a million followers who has no nutrition and health background, but gives those millions of followers advice that could, in fact, harm them. Everyone has the right to do as they wish and how they wish. But the damage it creates as far as how women or men should be perceived is unrealistic, and can cause severe psychological issues to those who don't know better. How do you think that is affecting the younger generations who see that? Are they obtaining a positive, happy feeling whenever they see women with hour-glass figures and fake implants in bikinis that barely cover anything? Or are they getting insecure because they don't look like that? How about young men? How do they feel when they see a nineteen-year-old adult with perfect abdominals and tight muscles?

Some will say that's inspiring, as it "motivates" them, yet a large group of others—who won't admit it—will probably feel like, at the age of thirty, they'll never look like as good as that. The result is a generation of people doing what I did in my past, and sadly, only worrying about the exterior. I've witnessed people go to the hospital because they injected oils into their arms to make them appear bigger. You read that right: oil injected into the arms to make them seem bigger. As I was at the airport returning home from a business expo, I remember clearly a seventeen-year-old kid looking at me, and I felt like he wanted to talk to me. His parents had gone to buy some food and he was there on his own.

As I smiled, he opened up and said he wanted to ask me a few questions. I'll never forget one of the questions he had for me. He explained that he'd always been the "bigger" student in the classroom, and he didn't know what to think about that. He followed that with asking whether I knew some of the people in the fitness industry. He named a few people, and I told him I knew them all. He then wondered if it would be okay to ask another question, but one that was more personal. He wanted to know if the people he'd brought up in our conversation were naturally gifted athletes, or if they had taken any performance-enhancing drugs.

I didn't feel like replying to the question, because what others tell me is confidential; however, I did tell him those types of drugs wouldn't help him because I knew the next question would be toward that subject. As I'd suspected, that was exactly his question. He further explained that a few of his friends in high school were taking pro-hormones (designer steroids), and that he was thinking about taking them, too. I spent almost an hour speaking to him, and I couldn't have been happier to do so. I made it clear that what he believed he saw on social media wasn't always entirely true, and secondly, there was no need to buy those illegal substances to get in shape, as he had everything he already needed to make his goals a reality.

Think about what that does to someone's level of happiness, seeing something on a small screen and then seeing their reflection in the mirror that's nothing alike. I'll speak more later on how to motivate yourself from *within*, and not from what you see. There's also the issue of athletes who spend hours editing their pictures with filters, Photoshop, and God knows what other ways, to look perfect in front of your eyes. I've asked you before to think about the people you follow on social media. Why do you follow them? A majority of us will say entertainment. I can see that. Many accounts are, indeed, funny, and they do entertain us. But the truth is that we follow those we seek to resemble. Can they inspire us to be better?

Honestly, I believe they only do in that one moment we see their photos. The next day I doubt you'll even remember what inspired you about their photo, because you'll have new photos to look at. I do not believe that a single photo has the power to motivate you for a lifetime, and that's what you constantly need to see they are doing. Additionally, the personality you assume they have is the personality they *want* you to believe. So when you combine nice clothes, fancy cars, and nice bodies, you are sucked into believing all those factors go hand in hand with success, thus creating the idea that you need those things in life, which makes you want to follow someone who already has them.

Realistically, the people you follow do have one thing you can do as well: work out. We start thinking that having a nice body will lead to fancy clothes, to perhaps a better home, and a better quality of life. Finally, these influencers then want to try and sell you a fitness program, because once again, you believe you too can do what they're doing if you follow their routine. Hopefully all of this makes sense to you. You need to realize that your happiness is under your control. Don't allow what you see to change your state of mind and then affect you negatively.

Don't seek hope and happiness in others or through others' social media platforms, as that's when these types of accounts will suck you in. I'm not being a hater or being negative; I myself have close to a million followers on my Facebook fan page. I'm trying to explain to you the process that's created when you base your thought process on what you see in other's posts. What happens when you follow the routine you bought from them—the one that promised a whole new you—and you don't reach those goals? You go on to try the next program and the next. Your level of happiness drops and you feel bad about yourself and your situation. Don't let that happen. Control your happiness by knowing that you have control over your life, and you have the necessary tools you already need to become happier on a daily basis.

I'm not saying all accounts and influencers are bad. I do not want you to believe that. I myself follow some incredible coaches on social media who constantly provide educational content. My message is for you to understand that fitness and happiness sold to you via the imagery of big muscles and big butts isn't going to ultimately provide what you want, which is to feel happy and confident. Remember what I said before about transformations that don't begin in the mind? First you must change your level of confidence and your state of mind before you can believe that the external person you are working for will do it for you.

Use social media to entertain you, and depending on who you follow, learn a few things. Have that potentially propel you to become more curious, and research topics you don't know about. Learn. As I said, I follow certain people because they honestly *do* care, and put out valuable, interesting content. Unfortunately they don't get the recognition they deserve, but most times these people aren't on social media with the intention of getting recognition. They are truly there to help those who want to read and learn from their posts.

These types of accounts and influencers will post topics and photos that aren't about them. They are trying to educate others with intellectual facts and research. How can you spot these genuine accounts? They aren't making their posts all about themselves—and *only* themselves. Their posts are about teachings and philosophies. Studies and research. They go against the current of the stream that everyone else is following. You, too, can share your story and inspire others. Don't allow the number of followers you have to affect you. If one person changes their life because of your story, then you've already changed the fate of one human: #letsmovemore.

- Don't always believe the hype you see from media outlets. Use social media to help you learn from those who teach, not show off.
- Don't allow your emotions to be altered by what others have already accomplished. If you already think you can't do it, you've already lost the battle.
- Share your story. Others, too, can relate to how hard life can be. Share the ways you've gotten to where you are so that others can learn from your life hacks and be motivated by you.

CHAPTER 11

FIND AND KEEP YOUR MOTIVATION: PART I

It always seems impossible until it's done.

—Nelson Mandela

've done seminars, talks, and made several posts on the subject of motivation, and it's one of those topics I still get questioned about the most. Motivation is a subject I could probably write an entirely different book about, and still have something new to add to it. Weekly I get someone at the gym asking me how I do it. How have I kept the light burning for so many years? Throughout this chapter we will analyze and discuss what motivation *is*, how to keep it, and most importantly, how to find your own. You might not be thinking about it as you read, but you're already working on increasing your motivation if you simply just think about it.

Before you read further, I want to make sure you know the difference between motivation and inspiration. We use these words interchangeably all the time, but there is a world of difference between the two. It's hard to be inspired daily, to have something so great within us that nothing will stop us from reaching our goals.

But you don't just get inspired, and then go from there. You use different techniques and forms of motivation to keep you going in reaching your ultimate inspiration.

The way I see it, inspiration is the ultimate desire or object you want to reach, and motivation comes from achieving the small goals that will get you there. It's hard to stay motivated all the time, and even harder to be inspired all the time. Life gets in the way, and our motivation for our inspiration can decrease. The key is understanding that you'll need to constantly motivate yourself in order to reach your goals. Just like it is with happiness—don't wait for it to happen. Create it.

Now that you know how to find your fit, you need to be able to stick with it. You need to be able to want to keep yourself motivated and inspired to do this in order to reach your goals. Here's the obstacle many people encounter: Their motivation isn't strong enough to get them out of bed, to make better decisions, and to push the extra five minutes during that hard exercise routine. As I said before, motivation won't just pop up out of nowhere. You have to be able to create a state of mind and sustain it. What's seriously going to make you want to push yourself daily? Hopefully it's not the last doctor's appointment you went to, where they said it was time to take care of your health or otherwise your health would suffer. If it *is* that, then now you have a wakeup call.

You know by now that trying to just look good won't be enough. It might motivate you for a bit, but it will not sustain long-term inspiration. You will need a deeper reason than that. You can say "I want to look good naked"—a superficial reason—but you will need something more personal to keep the wheel spinning. Let's take a step backwards. What does motivation even mean to you? Is it a special feeling? An emotion or thought you carry? Only you can define what your motivation means, and the level it can impact you.

Many believe that motivation is simply going to hit you like a bolt of lightning does. I've got bad news for you. Lighting only hits one in 960,000 people. Actually, that's a good thing! (You get the point!) Don't wait for motivation to strike you. Create your own. I do believe another person's energy and motivation can be transferred to you, the same way that watching your favorite YouTube video or podcast will do the same. But are you going to be watching videos or hanging out with those people for all of your life? Probably not.

Seeking motivation from social media can also be tricky. One moment you feel it, and then another you don't. What if you found out that your favorite fitness model routinely Photoshopped their photos? How would that make you feel, and would you trust any other fitness model you saw on social media? Could you gather motivation now from that source, knowing there's a big potential it's fake? As I mentioned earlier, the illusion of happiness is a great marketing scheme for anyone wanting to attract people to their products. The important thing is not where you obtain motivation from, but can you sustain it for long enough to get you moving and acting upon your goals?

The most successful millionaires probably didn't make their money over the course of their lifetimes by investing in only one source. You should do the same. Invest in different techniques and sources of motivation. Whether that's reading books in the morning, watching videos in the evening, or listening to music during your workouts. You need to use whatever it takes to keep your ball rolling. Imagine your motivation is the battery on your smartphone. You charge it a few times during the day, and also at night, so when you wake up your phone is fully charged. That's how your motivation should work.

Have a strong thought or feeling that you carry with you as your foundation, along with smaller ones you can use as an energy boosts. This can tremendously help you before going to work out, especially if you already imagine how that workout will look like, and how it's going to make you feel accomplished afterwards. I've used this technique myself several times whenever I've felt unmotivated to go train. That song or that video you use to get you pumped up, that's the perfect time for it, as it will get you moving. Moving is the key, and once you act on something without putting too much thought into it or analyzing it, you will get going.

I remember the days when I didn't want to even see a dumbbell. I was too tired to move due to the lack of proper nutrition, and it was the second workout of the day. I would sit in my car and have to watch something to get me feeling motivated. If I was even 1 percent better, I'd get out of the car and immediately walk through those gym doors. Just *act*. Do not think. Go. You will need something stronger for those snowy or rainy days, those days where you simply don't want to get out of bed. That's where your true motivation needs to kick in and outweigh any discouraging factors.

When I say "kick in," I don't mean you should wait around for something to happen. I'm saying you need to create the mental environment you need in order to get going. Turn the music up, move out of bed or off the couch, start getting dressed, and fill your water bottle. You might feel sluggish at first, but you aren't just thinking about it. You are acting on it at this point, and the likelihood of getting it done has dramatically increased. It's a lot easier for your brain to want to create a negative scenario or environment than it is to create one that's going to benefit you. It's simple, subconscious survival.

Another technique I can share with you, one that I know has helped many people, is visualization. Visualize something while you are listening to your favorite motivational song or video. The power of an image inside your heard plus the emotions of happiness, drive, excitement, etc., will create a stronger force inside of you than simply just imagining it without the addition of that emotion.

For men reading this book, if you have watched the move *Rocky*, do you remember that moment where he's going up those stairs? What made that scene so inspirational? It was a combination of music and exercise, and you visualizing yourself in his shoes.

"Eye of the Tiger" isn't just a song that became popular due to some random scene in the movie. It became popular because it was attached to a specific moment in the movie where Stallone was exercising and training to improve himself while defying struggles and odds. That's what you need to create for yourself every time you feel unmotivated to go exercise. For the ladies, it's the same concept. I want you to stop and visualize the scenes from *G.I. Jane*, *Flashdance*, or *Footloose*. They all incorporate songs of empowerment. When you feel the power in you, then you will want to take action. Yes, you read that right. Feel the power! Just like He-Man as he swings his sword in the air and says, " I have the power!"

By now you've probably gathered that I'm a fan of '90s action movies and cartoons. But as silly as it sounds, that's what you'll need to do every time you don't feel like exercising or making any positive choices in your life. When it comes to creating better habits, however, this technique might not be the best. When you're in public trying to make a decision between the grilled chicken salad or the cheesy macaroni, you might not feel so comfortable after screaming, "I have the power!" while swinging your fork in the air.

For occasions like these, where you know what you *should* do goes against what you are feeling would taste the best, I encourage you to not think about it too much. Immediately order the chicken salad as fast as you can. If you keep reading the menu to see what your options are, you might fall prey to the temptation to order something you shouldn't. If you are going to wait and see what your friends or family members are eating, you'll also be under social pressure as well. I am going to suggest two things: Don't ask others what they're going to order, and don't *tell* others what you'll be having either. If anyone asks just say you don't know, and when the server comes, just tell him. I don't know why people feel the need to know what others are eating, but the following sort of scenario is pretty typical.

Me: Menu looks great. Lots of options.
Friend: Yes! The french fries and the burger sound great! What are you getting?
Me: The tuna-steak salad.
Friend: Really?! You look good, man. You can afford to eat a burger, too. C'mon!

This happens every time I go eat with friends. People reaffirm that I look good, and that I should get a break from my lifestyle choices. It's not a diet; it's my lifestyle. Just because someone else can't be disciplined, doesn't mean you shouldn't be. In addition, *I'm* the one eating it, not the others at the table, so what does it matter what I get? The scenario above is common, and you need to realize that people want you to subconsciously make the same poor choices they are because they have no self-control. It makes them feel bad about themselves when you're eating something that's helping you toward your goals, while they are not. It can remind them, too, of what they should be doing, and aren't.

Making choices in situations like this has to be like having a sticker at the back of your mind. Put a backdrop on your phone that reminds you of your motivation. Remind yourself at all times, especially during the hard times, why you are doing what you are doing. Don't allow your motivation to suffer because others don't have it. The more frequently you make the right choices for yourself, the easier it is to re-wire your brain to keep making positive choices down the line.

• • •

I've often been told that people believe those who work out daily and wake up early must be different; they're either extremely motivated in life or they simply aren't normal. If normality means being lazy, hitting the snooze button ten times, and making poor health choices, then I don't want to be normal. The motivation I had at eighteen and my motivation now are completely different, and I'm no different than you or anyone else. The "secret" is something that I will share with you, and only you: It's called "Get off your lazy butt and go do it." There is no secret, yet thousands of trainers and social media people will tell you they have the ultimate secret to becoming a better you. Don't fall for that.

For me, it's simply a habit now. At first it wasn't a healthy habit, as you read earlier, but I turned it into something I can now use to my benefit. It's as much a habit for me as brushing my teeth and drinking water during the day. I do understand that this habit isn't for everyone. I, too, get lazy. I, too, want to sometimes stay home and order pizza and watch Netflix. Yet my source of motivation and inspiration is simple. I want to take care of the only body I was given. It's the only health I have, and the only shell that moves me on a daily basis. My main inspiration is to feel good about my body and mind.

My motivation comes from different, small sources, and I too need to constantly refresh and renew them. If that's not simple enough motivation for anyone, then I don't know what else to tell you. You are what your habits are. Plain and simple. As Harvard psychologist Jerome Bruner once said, "You are more likely to act yourself into feeling, than feel yourself into action." So move! Thinking about something is great, but if you don't take action than you're just a thinker, not a doer. That's why I emphasize that even just moving a little—even if it isn't the full action you need to take to reach your goal—is already a start.

Your body simply does what your mind believes it should do. The flipside to this is that if you allow your mind to overthink it, then you won't act either. There's a small amount of space for you to simply go and take action; otherwise, you'll suffer from what I call "thinker procrastination." You'll keep finding reasons, ways, and excuses to not do something. If your mind believes you aren't good enough, then that's what your body will believe, and you won't act. So for one second—just one—think to yourself what it would feel like to actually do what you thought. Start simple. It doesn't need to be complicated. That's the problem for most of us; we want to complicate things from day one, and not break it down to simple, obtainable objectives. As you progressively act, you will slowly build that habit.

Let's be honest, when I was eighteen, my motivation to train wasn't about being healthy. It was to look good. What teenager goes to the gym seeking health and happiness? They go to the gym because they're looking to attract the opposite sex. But even between the ages of eighteen and nineteen my motivation changed, in a matter of just one year. From that day onward, I only sought to better myself for the next time I'd step onstage again. From the age of twenty-two, when I turned into a professional athlete, I sought bigger things, and my motivation kept changing. Now, my goal is to inspire and help others find their own motivation and inspiration. My motivation now is completely different.

My foundation of motivation and inspiration back then is no longer the same today. You must understand that, since, as you evolve, the things that motivated you even yesterday might not motivate you today. Seeking your inner motivation now will require you to develop and grow. How do you do that? We change, we grow, we adapt, and we learn. The process then repeats itself. The first step I encourage you to take whenever you can't find motivation, is to spend some time by yourself.

Sit down and close your eyes. At first, all the things you did for that day will come to mind. Then all your problems will probably come into play. Finally, after you've been sitting for a while and you're breathing slowly, you will be able to focus on the task. Ask yourself, "What motivates me?" Think of the things you enjoy. Why do you enjoy them? If you are seeking motivation to go to the gym, then ask yourself, "Is my longevity on this earth not important to me? Is my family not important to me? Is how I feel on a daily basis not important to me?" These are simple, foundational questions.

You need to ask yourself what it is that's so strong, it will motivate you to do something out of your comfort zone. Bruce Springsteen said, "A time comes when you need to stop waiting for the man you want to become, and start being the man you want to be." The "man you want to be" needs to be the reason and motivation for you to do things outside of your comfort zone. Remember that the longer you wait to do something you should be doing now, the greater the odds that you will never actually do it—the Law of Diminishing Intent. But this is all easier said than done, I know. I've been through it.

Going to the gym almost every day for a decade made things a bit boring. So what did I do? I changed my entire fitness routine, and that itself made me want to seek motivation by learning not only how to perform new types of routines, but to also slowly get better at them. My overall inspiration was to become an overall better athletic individual, and my motivation came from simply vi-sualizing myself being good at the new exercises. Now I'm training to run my first Spartan race, something I have never done but is so outside my comfort zone that it sparks a fire for me to want to be good at it.

I know I won't be the best the first time I do it, but the second time I will be even more motivated, because I'll know how to further prepare myself. That's the thing about motivation. It changes. It transforms, and it keeps you moving. I believe a soul without inner motivation is a dead soul. That's the definition of a zombie to me: someone who is dead on the inside but alive on the outside.

- Motivate yourself daily with different resources so you can create the state of mind to act on your desired goals.
- What does motivation mean to you? Truly think about it, and then write down the things that motivate your inspiration. Think of at least three different things if you can, and place them somewhere you will be able to see them daily.
- Empower yourself with music, videos, emotions, etc. When you don't feel like doing something, don't think about it too much. Just act. The motions will enable you to get going.

FIND AND KEEP YOUR MOTIVATION: PART II

Your vision will become clear only when you look into your heart. Who looks outside, dreams. Who looks inside, awakens.

—Carl Jung

Your motivation is yours—no one else's. What motivates you shouldn't necessarily have to motivate others. Let me share a thought with you: Don't force your motivation on others. If both you and your partner are trying to lose weight, then you each need your own source of motivation to propel you toward your similar end goal. When it came to my clients, I would always ask them on our first day together what motivated and inspired them. Most didn't see the difference between the two, and that's fine. Once again, I'm not going to force something on them, but it was important for me to know what truly motivated them to take the right actions when I was not around.

Most of them wanted to lose the excess weight they'd put on as a result of their current lifestyles, so we would discuss that, and what ambitions they had in life. Sadly, many just lived day to day without any goals, ambitions, or desires, but this was an excellent chance to introduce fitness into their lives. Changing a lifestyle can be challenging. It takes time and dedication. Once you've finished the book, you'll have all the tools you truly need to make that change yourself. That's what motivated me to write this book for you. Motivation is as unique as the finger prints on your hands. Just because two people might be motivated by the same ideals does not mean they see that motivation the same way. That's why keeping your motivation and inspiration close to your heart and to yourself is important, because people like to take that away from others. I hate to say it, but that's human nature to do so.

I can't tell you how many times when I was young that I heard people tell me I was dreaming when I told them I was going to be at the Olympia stage one day, have sponsors backing me, and have multiple international fitness magazine covers. They smirked at me, they spoke behind my back, and they told me I would never be able to do all that. That was my motivation. That was all I needed—to prove them wrong. The fire would always spark in me when I was tired, sleepy, or unmotivated after I told myself I hadn't reached my goals and not going to the gym or eating the right meals wasn't getting me any closer to my destination. I turned everyone's negative energy into my positive energy. Today, no one—and I mean, *no one*—ever questions me when they ask what's next. They know what I am capable of. Now it's your turn to show others what you are capable of doing.

My desires would flame my motivation and keep me going but have you ever wondered why the majority of people don't lose weight or gain the muscle they want, even though that's what they desire the most? Does this sound familiar to you? January 1 comes around, and you start making your New Year's resolution. Then you start thinking about the goals you want to accomplish in January. You wish for it, just as you would if you saw a shooting star. Sometimes you even visualize it. On even rarer occasions, you write it down on a piece of paper so you're reminded daily of what you wished for.

You get motivated! You buy new shoes, new clothes, and start a new membership at a gym. The first two weeks you've lost a few pounds, and now you're more determined than ever to keep going. It feels amazing, since it's all new at that point. Then, by February, you feel like you're running at 65 percent capacity. Not at 100 percent. By March, the new shoes aren't new. The new clothes aren't new, and the new gym you thought was amazing the first time you went, is just another gym. What happened?! What changed in your mindset that made you—in less than three months—lose the original desire to change?

This also applies to anything in life in general, whether it's people seeking new relationships or new jobs with the idea in mind that such a change will be what they need to spark a new life. We enjoy novelty in our lives because it makes us feel good and excited. There's a part of our brain, in fact, that makes us feel like we're getting rewarded by all this novelty in and around our lives. But once the routine is done, things aren't new anymore, and possibly soon, you won't lose the weight you originally started losing because you aren't pushing yourself as much as you did in the beginning. Your nutrition isn't as healthy either, and you feel like something is missing, but you don't know what.

It's normal to feel like this. You're not the only one. We seek that feeling of new in several aspects of our lives: our relationships, our homes, our jobs, new clothes, and much more. The excitement goes away and everything feels stagnant. So how do we change that even after we've started working on our daily habits to improve ourselves slowly? It all begins in your mind. Those feelings of lacking motivation can be changed immediately. Have you taken the time to look at where you are now, currently—the choices you take, the actions you perform, and the mindset you've built? These things are all responsible for how you feel, perceive, and live life.

Just because something isn't new doesn't mean it's not working anymore for you. That's how you've made yourself perceive it. You don't need go out and buy new clothes or join a new gym. All you have to do is change your perceived notion of what you are already doing. Small things, like even completely changing your music playlist, can impact how you feel. If you like running or walking outside, then change the path a bit. Go look at some new scenery.

A question that helped me through those phases was, "Who do I want to be? Not *what* do I want to do, but who do I want to be—for myself?" In my mind I used to picture the "perfect" physique. That's all! That was my ambition in life. Pretty poor, huh? Then, as life changed, so did my ambitions. If you aren't happy with your current situation, it's most likely because you aren't living the life you want. To change that you need to immediately change your ways of thinking. Then ask yourself that same question again: "Who do I want to be?" Do you want to be healthier, more generous, more loving, more ambitious, more patient?

Secondly, you need to ask yourself, "What can I do right now to change my state of mind so I can change my perception of life?" What actions can you take to get there? Staying physically active will help you with your health and your physique. There's honestly unlimited actions you can take right now that will help you grow to be slightly healthier every day. Don't tell yourself that because you aren't in the gym and because you aren't eating vegetables for all your meals that there isn't something you could be doing to be healthier today.

We tend to associate discomfort with anything that's new to us. That's the biggest problem right there. When we think about weight loss, we immediately think of diets, and diets aren't fun. They require discipline. But what if you were to re-wire that thought process, and instead think diet *equals* weight loss, and weight loss equals a better life? It means more energy to go play ball with a few friends or to go out dancing with the girls. Don't make the association that the media has created for you, because that's how they will win.

They know that when you think of weight loss you think discomfort and pain, so what do they do? They create ads with people who are happy in life, telling you their product will make you not feel hungry, sad, or depressed about your current situation. Re-wire your thought process when it comes to things you don't take immediate pleasure in doing. Drinking more water is one the easiest things you could be doing to help your health, and it doesn't require that much effort or action. In return, you will feel better, more confident, and more energized. The better you feel, the more hooked on that feeling you'll become, and the more actions you will take to remain or improve not only your health, but all aspects of your life. See how it's all related?

Do you still need more motivation to improve your health? Get committed, and don't depend on others. Don't allow what I'm going to tell you next to prevent you from reaching out to people you feel can help—but don't depend on them to strike. In my own journey I haven't had much luck finding a mentor. Every single self-help book preaches that in order to be successful you must find a mentor or reach out to others with experience, someone who's already walked the walk and knows the ways of reaching your desired success.

I remember reaching out to a good amount of people to whom I could potentially contribute ideas and share my thoughts with. These were not people out of my reach, either. These were individuals I knew personally at one point or another, who I'd had conversations with in person, so it wasn't like I was trying to reach out to the president of the United States for financial advice or to

Tony Robbins for advice about life. Sadly, only one person wrote back, and unfortunately they told me they didn't have time for me. Disappointed by this, I l realized that I would have to be my own mentor, and learn things on my own.

Needless to say, that didn't mean I stopped attempting to reach out to others. But it *was* a realization that mentors these days aren't what most books from twenty or thirty years ago make them out to be. The lesson of this story is that I had to start moving forward on my own in order to create my own success. I do know one thing for a fact. It's the people who take action in the world who are the ones who create their own success. So if you don' know what to do in a gym facility, just start moving on a treadmill or cardiovascular machine that you feel comfortable doing. If you're financially able to, hire a trainer. Research them first.

As you keep training or working out in any sport of your liking, either research people in your area who are good at what they do, or talk to them. See how they like to approach helping people individually based on their own goals. This will keep you accountable, and will motivate you. During my years training, I realized that some of my clients had the full power to go to the gym on their own, but they preferred having me there to keep them accountable for going and pushing them. This is a great way to keep you moving forward. Remember, even if you are crawling to your destination, you are still moving forward. Movement is life!

Ralph Waldo Emerson said, "Whatever course you decide upon, there is always someone to tell you that you are wrong." A big component of your motivation is your environment. Who you surround yourself with, who your friends are, what they mainly talk about, and your environment at home can facilitate your motivation or complicate it. Remember that you are accountable for all the choices you make in life, and that includes your surroundings. Choices, in case you happened to forget, are actions and thoughts we take once something or someone acts upon our lives.

If you made the choice to surround yourself with negative people, then you always have the ability to act and change that. Even if it's your best friend or family member, if they are not contributing to an atmosphere that allows you to become a better version of yourself, then it will be a challenge to maintain a sky-high level of motivation. Forget about your inspiration, then. If you have no energy to stay motivated, then eventually your inspiration will vanish, too. You have full control over the food you buy and bring home. If someone buys the food for you, then you need to make the necessary choice to begin going to the store yourself, and making wiser choices to help you in your goals.

Your atmosphere and what you surround yourself with at home can dramatically affect you. If all you bought were snacks, junk food, and unhealthy meals, then why would you ever think it's possible to lose weight? You are not creating the atmosphere you need to stay on track. If all your friends go to happy hour after work and are barely involved in any physical activity, then why would you want to be any different? You need to make an effort to change the atmosphere you are surrounded by. This will, in turn, affect your motivation, your thoughts, and your feelings, which will lead you to making better choices.

Making new friendships is sometimes a must. If you feel no one around you is contributing to your choices, or even making them more complicated, then it's time to change your friendship environment. Many people meet their loved ones at gyms, and many in fact build whole new networks and friendship circles at the gym. Why can't you? Let me share with you the story of one of my former clients. He was an overweight, middle-aged, divorced man. He'd just gone through his divorce a few months prior and wanted to get back in shape, as he felt the divorce had taken a lot out of him. I could relate to him on the matter of divorce, but I needed to show him that life wasn't over because of it.

He told me he wanted to lose twenty pounds, which is the amount he'd gained in the few months post-divorce. As I got to know him session by session, I realized he had become a very lonely and somewhat shy person. He told me his wife took away all their mutual friendships, along with their two children, and he now lived in a small condo because that's all he could afford at the time. It's a very common story. His optimistic feelings toward whether he would ever fit in again anywhere were shattered, no doubt. His only social hours would be spent with me or with a few coworkers he'd meet after work for happy hour. From what he expressed, however, he felt like his coworkers only allowed him to tag along because they felt bad for him.

I told him this: "We need to change your life *now*—not tomor-row—NOW!" I also said he needed to do a few things to turn his life around. First, he needed to stop feeling sorry for himself. Divorces happen, and life isn't fair. But the first thing he needed to change was his friendships, his atmosphere at home, and the way he perceived life. His entire atmosphere needed to change if we were going to improve his motivation, not only in respect to his health— which at that point was on a path to disaster—but his motivation and inspiration for life.

Read carefully, as you can do these things yourself and apply them to any area of your life. First, you need to realize that the world will not stop because of you. We all feel like we are the center of the universe, that our problems are the biggest, and that life won't ever be the same because we can't fix these problems. In order to do this, you need to also realize that you, like any other person out there, have the power and the choices to change your life *now*. Many believe that those people who are meant to succeed are "special." They're not! They make the choice they need to change.

Second, you need to change your thought process. If all you

can think about is how something bad is going to happen next, then guess what—it will, and you'll miss out on all the positive things around you, too. The longer you procrastinate, the longer these issues will continue to linger in your head. But as I said, the world keeps on moving, and so do you. By changing the way you think, you can change how you perceive these problems, and you'll understand that life will always have problems to throw your way.

Third, take action to resolve those problems. Thinking about them all day won't solve anything. If anything, that will result in a panic attack. Clients come to me all the time with their problems, and as they share them, I'm automatically thinking of ways to fix them. Be a problem solver, not a problem sharer. When I'd share my thoughts about possible solutions, they would find more excuses to not solve the problems. Sometimes, a complicated problem has, indeed, a very simple solution—just like in my client's case, who felt the world was over because of his divorce.

What he failed to realize is that by hiring me he had already taken a huge step forward. He had taken his first step into action to improve his life, and improve the circumstances that he felt were tormenting him. Take an initial step; join a gym, buy new gym clothes if you can, join a fitness class, or hire a certified trainer. If these are the small actions you need to get motivated, then do them. Don't just think about doing them. Surround yourself with like-minded people who want to be at the gym or taking part in any outdoor recreational activity. These are people who most likely will become your new friends if you keep showing up.

That's exactly what happened with my client. After being there for over a month, he told me he'd met two guys who had seen him training with me and they'd asked if he wanted to join them for a quick lunch. He accepted, and told me all about it. I felt like a dad hearing his son talk about this exciting new game or toy he had. He was so happy that day that he'd forgotten about his shyness, and made two new friends. He later asked if it was okay for him to work out with one of the guys he'd met, and I was all for it. Eventually I told him he needed to make initial conversation of his own, the same way those two men had approached him. Not only for that reason, but to also potentially talk to new women at the gym, so he'd no longer feel like there was no one who would ever like him.

As he progressed with me, he lost thirty pounds, and he felt like a whole new man, not because he'd lost thirty pounds, but because he'd gained a new insight in his life. He had forgotten all his past reasons that were inhibiting him from moving forward, and he completely changed his environment. It wasn't just the physical aspect that had changed, but his entire persona was completely different. His clothes changed, the way he walked and stood changed, the way he spoke about himself changed, and his habits had changed, too—all because he took a small risk at hiring a trainer. Even though he had no idea that was an accomplishment, he'd done that on his own. The power of people who surround you, along with a new place to exercise, think, and live can make enormous changes in your life. The change, however, must come from you *knowing* something must change in order for you to make progress and for your motivation to sky rocket.

Finally, one of the biggest reasons most people are unmotivated is because they see the end result of other people's hard work, and they mentally talk themselves out of even starting. Not starting any type of action due to comparison is automatic suicide. That's why you need to learn to choose the right things with which you associate yourself. This applies to what you choose to look at as well. Whether it's your friends with whom you like to compare yourself, or the models on social media who may have Photoshopped their pictures to look completely unrealistic, remember to never compare your own journey with someone else's. You don't know how long that person has been doing what they've been doing, the huge amounts of sacrifice it took for them to get there—or potentially even the illegal substances they might have taken to look like that, compromising their health along the way.

Most fitness magazine covers are full of edits. Did you know a cover can take a few to several hours in a day just to get that one magical shot? Even the best models in the world spend hours, because they truly want that picture to be out of this world. You also don't know what magical tweaks were made on the computer to highlight and/or hide certain features. If you feel depressed just looking at those images and tell yourself you can't improve things, it only means one thing. You need to work on your self-esteem, and most importantly, you need to stop looking at things that make you feel negatively about yourself. Immediately! You shouldn't associate yourself with anything that makes you feel self-doubt. Low self-esteem is what will keep you where you currently are, and it won't provide you with the energy to want to propel yourself forward.

So why do many people have low self-esteem and fail to realize their full potential, when we all have the power to be great? This is question that you'll need to sit down in a quiet area, do some self-reflection, and think about. Often it starts from childhood: how you were raised and how you felt about yourself growing up, among other things. But these can all be changed. Worrying about what others think of you won't pay your bills, won't make you happier, and definitely won't help you take action in your life. Someone's thoughts about you should never define who you are unless you allow them to have that power. If anything, use those thoughts to propel you forward. Use their negative statements and turn them into energy like I did.

Just take a good look in the mirror. Look yourself in the eye, and finally realize that nothing is going to change unless you take action to change it. If third-party sources, like social media, friends, and even family, make you feel less than what you're worth, it's time to eliminate those elements, or slowly reduce their presence in your life. That's right! Family, too! Family can be one of the hardest things to deal with. Just because your voice bounces around inside your brain doesn't mean you have to listen to it. Eventually you'll find a more positive energy source, but if that's what initially gets you going and grinding, then so be it. The only person who will ever make you feel unmotivated is *you*.

- Convert the negative energy around you into positive energy. Transform your mindset so that every time a negative statement comes out of someone else's mouth, you utilize it as a positive, propelling force.
- Start re-wiring your thought process so that every time you think of something that brings you discomfort, whatever it is becomes something that brings you happiness and pleasure. Diets don't need to equate to being hungry and tired. Change your perspective so you can change the outcome.
- It's great to ask for help. In fact, I highly recommend it. But don't depend on others to achieve what you need to achieve. Accept help, if you must, to propel you forward faster, but you are the one who should always initially start the engine.
- You need to know something must change in order to change it. You can't just wish for new things in your life to happen if you don't know what those things are or how to approach them. If you want to lose weight, don't just point to the obvious and say, "I need to lose weight." Change your statement to, "I know I need to eat less junk food and exercise more. Let me sit down and make a plan for action."
- What do you feel is stopping you from taking action? Write down your thoughts on a piece of paper or in your smartphone, and figure out the why of why it is you believe you

can't do it. Here comes the important part of this bullet point: Beside each of those reasons you've just listed, write down the possible solutions to those problems. Money and time tends to be the most common reasons people believe they can't get in shape.

CHAPTER 13

TRIO OF HEALTH: THREE PILLARS

*As a rule, the mind, residing in a body that has become
weakened by pampering, is also weak, and where there is no
strength of mind there can be no strength of soul.*
—Mahatma Gandhi

The chest, biceps, and shoulders. No, those aren't the three pillars of health. But ask any guy at the gym and they'll probably say they are. The three pillars of health: your mind, body, and spirit. They have an equally balanced importance in your life, as they are all part of one great entity. From what I have seen and learned, most people have control over their bodies, but not so much when it comes to their mind and spirit. Personally, I struggled with my mind and spirit for years, and only after I stopped demanding so much from my body did I find equal force to add to the others. You can't expect to have all three in balance if you only put energy into one of those pillars. Ancient Greek and Chinese cultures already believed in these three pillars thousands of years ago, and how they could dramatically affect one's life and being. These cultures, and many others, believed in a life force that connected these three pillars. What does each pillar consist of, and what is its importance to your overall lifestyle?

Your mind. I'll start their, as I personally believe the mind is one of the hardest pillars to fully grasp. Your mind controls everything, from cognitive functions to capacities. In my opinion, it's the most important pillar of the three, and I would personally place it in the middle, between the other two pillars. Unfortunately, however, the mind is one aspect we think about least. Have you ever gotten a massage, practiced yoga, or done anything physically relaxing for your body? How did you feel afterwards? You mind sends signals to your body, and relaxes you physically when you create the environment to allow the mind to do its job.

When was the last time you *put thought* into your thoughts? The last time you sat down to analyze why you think the way you do? A healthy mind should be similar to your body, where you don't feed it junk. The same way you do a nutritional regimen to clean your body and feel better, your mind should also have a regimen of "clean" thoughts on a daily basis. The more negative thoughts and junk you feed the mind, the more it will become accustomed to it, and begin to automatically think that way. A completely healthy person who has a full grasp of their mind understands their thoughts and how they react to the events happening around them.

If you were to stop everything you're doing, put away your phone, sit quietly in a room, and start thinking about your thoughts, you'd learn a lot about yourself and the decisions you make. For example, if today you decided to go off your diet and eat a burger, when you shouldn't have made that decision, stop and think, *Why did I order that from the menu instead of staying on track?* Traditionally, however, we don't put that much thought into our thoughts, and we never really question ourselves about the things we're doing. To control our thoughts means to stop and make better, more rational decisions. A healthy mind can't be polluted by its environment.

As I mentioned earlier in the book, we spend so much time on social media watching videos and looking at pictures that we get polluted by other people's ideas of what we should look like. The consequence of this is that we feel differently about ourselves, and can lose that previous sense of well-being. By cleansing the mind, you are able to see past a negative environment or thought, and don't allow it to cloud the mind. As I said, though, the mind is one of the hardest things to keep healthy, as it is bombarded daily with new thoughts.

On average, most people have anywhere between fifty to seventy thousand thoughts in a day—an average of forty-eight thoughts per minute. It's nearly impossible to keep all of those thoughts positive, but how it impacts you is, without a doubt, controllable. The most successful people in the world will tell you that to keep a healthy mindset you should practice the act of meditation. I'm not going to go over the process of meditation, as you can look it over online or download an app to help you, but it's as simple as sitting down—before the day has started, ended, or anytime you feel overwhelmed—and then closing your eyes and breathing deeply through your nose and exhaling through your mouth.

Do this for ten minutes daily, and allow the process of your thoughts to roam free. How you decide to meditate is entirely up to you. I have been practicing this for over two years, and it simply makes me feel better. By feeling better, I've already had a positive start to my day. You should make a list of the things that calm you down and give you inner pleasure, as these are things you should practice daily. This doesn't mean going out and eating your favorite burger or pizza every day because it makes you feel good—that's you trying to fill the gap of happiness with food.

Slowly get into a morning ritual that makes you feel better as your day starts, whether that's watching your favorite influencer on social media who inspires you to be better (not just look better), listening to your favorite songs, or reading a quote from a book. Get into a habit of clearing your mind with positive thoughts or actions, and allow that to be your bridge to the start of your day. Often the first thing we do in the morning, as soon as our eyes open, is check our phones. You check your social media, your email, your texts, etc.

I can't tell you how many times I would start my morning upset after I allowed some comment on my social media affect me. Allowing energies from the outside to affect you is one aspect we all have to improve upon for a healthier mind. The same way you do squats for your legs to get stronger, practice the art of ignoring to strengthen the mind. A strong mind will always see the glass half full—not half empty. A strong mind will be able to push past any difficulties and limiting beliefs. A strong mind will be able to stay in control of itself, and will allow you to develop balance between it, your body, and your spirit.

Your spirit: Normally we hear about the mind and body, how well connected they are and how harmoniously both work together. Ever hear of the popular bodybuilding phrase "muscle-mind connection"? We don't hear the phrase "muscle-spirit connection." In fact, most people don't even think about that pillar when it comes to their health. You can use different words to describe this element, and many refer to this pillar as "the soul." The spirit is ultimately responsible for providing the body with its life force. Those who are religious are going to have an easier time identifying what this consists of, but those who aren't, don't worry.

You can think of the spirit as the bridge between the mind and body; a bridge that will connect your emotions and how you feel. Your spirit affects your mind, and vice versa. Emotional health is closely related to this pillar and you can also think of it as a connection to something greater than ourselves. I personally like to think of spiritual health as my motivation sometimes. Sure, the mind controls my motivation, inspiration, and my main emotions, but when something truly motivates me, I feel a certain way I can't even describe; there are no words for it. Have you ever felt that you were meant to do something? That inside of you—although you may not be able to describe it—you were meant to take certain action? It's almost like your gut is trying to tell you something.

That's how I perceive my spiritual connection. A healthy spiritual connection allows you to have faith in things you don't see. For example, you know deep down you'll be able to lose your ten pounds, even though you can't see it and emotionally your mind is telling you you're slightly unmotivated. Yet some greater force is making you feel like you know—you just *know*—those ten pounds will come off. That's how you should see all of this. Holistic healing can take great part in your spiritual health lifestyle, and more clinics are showing up these days that take this approach. They promote different services to relax you beyond just the physical, and they allow your mind to free itself so you can truly let go of everything around you. You almost feel cleansed of your problems, and your mind has the freedom to wonder. Meditation, again, is a great way to relax the mind and the spirit, which in turn, leads to better physical health.

Your body. To have a healthy body you must do your best to conquer a healthy mind. After all, any change starts mentally and then progresses physically. You will usually give up mentally before you give up physically. Our bodies and our physical health is partly determined by our mental health. Your body is the instrument given to you to move through this life. Have you ever noticed that when you don't exercise you feel tired and depressed more easily? That's your body affecting your mind. You only get one body, so you might as well take care of it. Unfortunately that statement doesn't really mean a lot to the millions of people who drink, smoke, do drugs, or, as with my past, only take care of the exterior. The mind at that point has lost the battle, and the body is paying the consequences.

The exterior needs to be balanced with the interior. Normally, if you take care of your internal self, the external self will have an easier time taking care of itself. What do I mean? If you eat the right foods in the right amounts, rest, hydrate, and exercise, then the exterior will be a showcase of all that. You can't expect to eat junk food, sleep little, never exercise, and overeat if you want to look like someone who's healthy. In fact, your body will show physical signs of it.

Drugs usually affect people's eyes, teeth, and even skin color, and so does drinking and smoking. The two best ways to keep your body healthy, as you might have already guessed, are through proper nutrition and exercise. These two combined will prolong your life and help with your spirit and mind. As you can tell by now, the mind, body, and spirit are all well connected, and they help one another to work at optimal, balanced capacity. You now know that a low percentage of body fat isn't always an indication of health. When you over-exercise and under-eat to get to 4-5 percent, your body is actually in survival mode.

Another example is someone who smokes, barely eats, and is constantly stressed. That individual might have a low body-fat percentage, but there's nothing healthy about it. Having a body that's healthy can mean many different things to different people, but in general it means a body that isn't ill or sick, has a good capacity for physical exercise, and a healthy internal organism. This should be one of the easiest of the three pillars to take care of, as you have full power of control over what you eat and how much you exercise.

Few can truly say they have mastered all three pillars. They are like three cards that form a pyramid, and you not only have to build them up slowly, but you have to build them with patience. Some days we feel like we have better control of our minds and bodies, but then there are days where we feel that our mind and spirit prevail. As easy as you may feel that you have control, you may suddenly feel that you've completely lost it. It just depends how easy you shatter. If you allow others to get in your thoughts and feelings, then your spirit and mind will always be weak. If you allow your emotions to get the best of you and you get lazy and don't exercise, then your body will suffer. One pulls on the other. That's why I feel it's extremely important that you create a habit of taking care of all three pillars of your health.

Set goals for each of the pillars. With time, no one or anything in your way will be able to make you crumble. Creating the necessary habits will also ensure that those three pillars are as balanced as they can be. Everyone works in different ways, and learning how you work and what works best for your lifestyle, will create the life you've been seeking. Take notes, perhaps, on what you see others doing for themselves, and then try them, applying your own style of approach.

CHANGE YOUR LIFE NOW

• • •

Use the following exercise to set goals for balancing and achieving the three pillars of health. Go back and look at this anytime you need to re-evaluate, create, and remind yourself of what needs to be done, and *how* it will be done, in order to improve your overall quality of life.

- **What are my goals?** (Is it to lose weight? Increase lean muscle mass? Be more active?) Write down your three most important desired goals.

    1.
    2.
    3.

- **Why haven't I reached my goals so far?** (<u>Be honest with yourself</u>. I can't help you if you don't help yourself first. Don't just write "time" or "money." If you do, then you need to dig deeper, because everyone can make the time to take care of themselves on some small level.)

    1.
    2.
    3.

- **How can I solve the above problems?** (Think of solutions to your above excuses.)

    1.
    2.
    3.

- **Why are my goals important to me?** (Write down the reasons these goals are important to you. If you don't have a true "why," then your chances of reaching your goals won't be high.)

    1.
    2.
    3.
    4.

- **What tools will I utilize daily to keep myself motivated to reach my ultimate inspiration?** (List at least five, as you can rotate them around. You can even use this book as one of them.)

    1.
    2.
    3.
    4.
    5.

- **What are five things I can do right now to start changing my body, mind, and soul?**

    1.

    2.

    3.

    4.

    5.

CHAPTER 14

BALANCE UNTIL THE END

*Happiness is not a matter of intensity but of balance
and order and rhythm and harmony.*
—Thomas Merton

Balance is never achieved until you fully understand it. To have a balanced life you must make it a priority to enjoy it and take care of it simultaneously. It's a complicated subject that can and will take time to incorporate into your life, but will make you a complete individual. So many things can throw us off, but just like a punching bag that takes on all of life's hits, you center yourself right back. When incorporating balance into your life, you must know what your priorities are; family, health, and work are usually what most people think of. If you were to break those apart even further, you would have even more priorities. I would highly encourage you to write down the things and people who matter to you in this life, that way you can visualize what needs to be balanced in your life, and you aren't left pondering what you believe should be worked on.

Whatever you write down must be of importance to you. Listing random things you wish were priorities won't help too much unless you start giving them purpose. Let's take your health, for example. If you haven't prioritized your health until you started reading this book, then you must fill out the previous goal sheet and give yourself a reason why it's now a priority. Family shouldn't need a reason, and most people already know why their jobs are important to them. Yet millions of people don't prioritize their health and fitness. Hopefully after reading this book you'll understand the important of including it as a priority.

Factors like time and stress are usually why people have a hard time balancing priorities, but if whatever it was, was indeed a priority they'd make time to do it. Money is then the driving force for most, and it blurs their vision of life. Just remember one thing: money comes and goes. Your health doesn't. Once you've damaged your body, mind, and spirit, it can be complicated to mold it back. Remember what I previously said about money. It's not going to provide you with the happiness you think it's going to, and I can speak from years of training people with a lot of wealth who couldn't balance health into their lives. You will need to create the time to incorporate all of the foundations in this book in order to succeed in your goals. No magic pill will save you the time; you must invest in yourself *now*.

Living with balance is crucial, and enjoying life is a must. Knowing that with balance you can enjoy and live a longer life should be the force driving you seek. Balance also means enjoying the things you like. That's why we say that everything in moderation is ideal. The eighty-twenty rule is a phenomenal way to approach most things. Stay on track 80 percent of the time, and enjoy the other 20 percent. This will enable you to balance the things you enjoy while always remaining guided with what we should be doing for our goals. We all need that 20 percent, as it is almost impossible to be running at full capacity all the time without crashing at one point or another.

Don't allow your 80 percent to be deviated by or stopped by anything or anyone but yourself. Put the little screen down once in a while and start appreciating the little things around you. Give yourself at least twenty minutes a day to work on yourself. Read, breath, or take more time and go work out. It's a necessity that you balance your goals in order to balance your thoughts, emotions, and feelings. Give your mind a chance to stay motivated on daily basis and create a life that you want to be involved in. The last thing you should want is to wake up and hate the day ahead of you. Balance also means creating a life you desire so that you control its outcome. After all, who else is the designer of your life but you? We tend to allow our balance to go off-kilter because of our self-induced problems. Most things that cause us stress are in fact either one of two things, both of which we have full control over. Either it's a matter of perspective, or it's a self-created problem. What do I mean?

In reality, problems are situations we haven't figured out yet how to solve, and that initially scares us as they float through our minds without order. Once you find a solution to a problem, when that same situation occurs you'll most likely know exactly what to do without stressing out. Sometimes there are multiple solutions to a problem and it's a matter of how you view it that will solve it. In other circumstances, we create a bigger problem than what it was initially, because we don't know how to manage our time and all the things you have to currently do—and the things you still have to do—become a big ball of thoughts that you can't unwind. That's when writing everything down helps you to visualize the tasks at hand.

As I said, most problems shouldn't be stressed over, but can be solved by solutions you just haven't thought of yet, or may need further organization. These techniques will help you balance whatever you think needs work. That's why it's crucial to take care of the mind, body, and spirit. Doing so will enable your entire system to operate smoothly and calmly without the added stress. From my experience, this absolutely works. I used to be a very stressed and unhappy individual all the time, and that's why I wasn't easy to deal with, especially in relationships. With time, self-work, and the help of others, I am much better at confronting situations so I'm able to balance the areas of my life as needed.

I want to finish this book by asking you the same questions I asked at the beginning. I want you to stop and think just for a few minutes about how you still perceive fitness and yourself. Ask yourself, "What is health? What do I want for my own health and life? How do I view health, and how do I feel about myself in this current moment?" I want you to fill out the goals sheet in the previous chapter with patience, and really think carefully about not only how you're going to solve your goals, but what they mean to you. As you now know, health can be viewed and interpreted in several different ways, but hopefully you have a better idea as to what you want out of your own health.

I want you to start developing the habits you will need to conquer anything you truly want to master. Remember, habits are just repetitive actions you take. Nothing else. Don't forget, we are humans after all, and it's in our nature to make silly mistakes— mistakes we slowly and hopefully learn from, and try to avoid repeating in the future. Don't live through others and what they might or might not be doing on social media. Create a real life for yourself. Losing the weight you want and improving your health are just one act away. Now is the time to take action. Now is the time to create a path to change your life. Don't believe that you have to be a victim of misfortune and bad luck to change your path in life.

I used to believe that my overweight clients needed a wakeup call or a tragedy to happen in order to see that their habits weren't going to lead them anywhere. But that's not true. If you can start seeing the good without anything bad, then you've already won half the battle. The key to fitting in the world and changing your life immediately is simple. Love yourself daily, and never self-doubt. Fit in with yourself first, and then you'll be able to master your health—and anything else you desire in life.

ABOUT THE AUTHOR

As an international leading fitness authority, Alexandre Carneiro has spent the last decade educating others on the meaning of fitness, health, and connecting those two things with a healthy mind. With a bachelor's degree in kinesiology and nutrition, along with positive, motivating philosophies, Carneiro has helped people all over the world achieve their fitness goals.

www.ingramcontent.com/pod-product-compliance
Lightning Source LLC
Chambersburg PA
CBHW070128260726
48658CB00001B/306